GETTING BETTER

GETTING BETTER

*Improving Health System Outcomes
in Europe and Central Asia*

Owen Smith
Son Nam Nguyen

THE WORLD BANK
Washington, D.C.

Contents

v

Boxes

Figures

Tables

Foreword

Recent years have brought economic turmoil to Europe and its
neighborhood, and the attention of policy makers has naturally been
drawn, even more than usual, to the ups and downs of their economies. This focus is justified: much will depend on charting a course
toward rapid recovery and sustained growth. But when we think
about the issues that will matter most to people in the region over a
longer horizon, other priorities come into sharper focus. From this
viewpoint, there are perhaps few challenges more compelling than
those facing health systems across the region.

There are at least two reasons to believe that health is a major
development challenge facing Europe and Central Asia (ECA) today.
First, looking back over several decades, we note that the region's
progress in health—as measured by indicators such as life
expectancy—has been among the slowest in the world. Instead of
catching up with Western Europe, many countries in the region have
been falling behind. Although recent years have seen some improvement, parity is still a long way off.

Second, looking forward, we see evidence that better health
becomes an increasingly important aspiration among populations as
countries grow richer. Aging societies will reinforce this trend.
Indeed, a joint EBRD-World Bank survey undertaken across the

region in both 2006 and 2010 indicated that health was consistently ranked the top priority for government investment among respondents in over three-quarters of the countries, including among men and women, young and old, rich and poor. Living long and healthy lives matters as much as achieving ever-higher incomes.

This book highlights three major agendas for health systems. First, health outcomes can be significantly improved—especially in the area of cardiovascular disease—in large part through wider implementation of cost-effective measures. Second, there is a need to ensure that better health care is financed in a way that does not impose an undue burden either on households or on governments. And third, the institutional arrangements that govern health systems must be strengthened by adopting some of the key ingredients common to advanced health care systems that are still absent in many countries in ECA.

The World Bank is refocusing its efforts to advance the development agenda with a view to end extreme poverty and promote shared prosperity. In the health sector, this will mean reducing large out-of-pocket payments for health care by households and extending access to high-quality health care services to the most vulnerable people. The ECA region can be proud of many achievements on both these fronts, but much still remains to be done. As World Bank President Jim Yong Kim has noted, "all of our clients are challenged by delivery—the design, execution and demonstration of results." Nowhere is this truer than in health care delivery, but the rewards for making progress will be enormous.

The health sector challenges described in this book are common to many other middle-income countries around the globe, and thus the key messages should resonate with audiences outside Europe and Central Asia. But above all, the book offers insights to policy makers in the region who seek to achieve a more prosperous and healthy future for their people.

Philippe Le Houérou	Ana Revenga
Vice President	Director, Human Development
Europe and Central Asia Region	Europe and Central Asia Region
The World Bank	The World Bank

Acknowledgments

The ECA regional health report "Getting Better" was prepared by a team led by Owen Smith and Son Nam Nguyen, under the guidance of Abdo Yazbeck and Daniel Dulitzky (sector managers, health) and Mamta Murthi and Ana Revenga (sector directors, human development). Background work and written contributions were also made by Rabia Ali and Ethan Yeh. Research assistance was provided by Courtney Chang, Nicole Cimbak, and Tatiana Voloh. The institutional characteristics survey presented in chapter 6 was implemented by a large number of World Bank staff and by the World Health Organization (WHO) European Observatory, led by Ewout van Ginneken, in collaboration with government counterparts serving as key informants.

This report is part of the Regional Study Program of the Europe and Central Asia Region of the World Bank, conducted under the leadership of the regional chief economist, Indermit Gill. The report team is grateful for the guidance and support of Indermit Gill and Willem van Eeghen throughout preparation of this study.

The report team is also grateful to numerous individuals who provided input and comments at various stages of the report's preparation. The team benefited from consultations with Michael Borowitz (Organisation for Economic Co-operation and Development [OECD]),

Maria Luisa Escobar, Josep Figueras (WHO European Observatory), Charles Griffin, April Harding, Joe Kutzin (WHO), Truman Packard, and all members of the ECA region's health team. Agnes Couffinhal provided detailed comments. Survey work was implemented in part with the support of the Bank-Netherlands Partnership Program (BNPP) and Global Alliance for Vaccines and Immunization (GAVI) trust funds. The team also gratefully acknowledges the comments of peer reviewers at both the concept note stage and the final review. The peer reviewers were Cristian Baeza, Enis Baris, Michael Borowitz (OECD), Charles Griffin, Daniel Kress (Gates Foundation), Truman Packard, and Agnes Soucat.

Lastly, the team would like to express its appreciation to Regina Nesiama for her assistance at many stages of the report's preparation; to Aziz Gökdemir, Paola Scalabrin, and Dana West for excellent production and editorial support; and to Elena Karaban, Dorota Kowalska, and Aarthi Sivaraman for their help with report dissemination.

Abbreviations

CIS	Commonwealth of Independent States (Armenia, Azerbaijan, Belarus, Kazakhstan, the Kyrgyz Republic, Moldova, the Russian Federation, Tajikistan, Turkmenistan, Ukraine, and Uzbekistan)
CPV	clinical performance and value
CT	computed tomography
CVD	cardiovascular disease
DRG	diagnosis-related group
EBRD	European Bank for Reconstruction and Development
ECA	Europe and Central Asia
EHIF	Estonian Health Insurance Fund
EU	European Union
EU-10	Bulgaria, Czech Republic, Estonia, Hungary, Latvia, Lithuania, Poland, Romania, Slovak Republic, Slovenia
EU-11	Bulgaria, Croatia, Czech Republic, Estonia, Hungary, Latvia, Lithuania, Poland, Romania, Slovak Republic, Slovenia
EU-15	Austria, Belgium, Denmark, Finland, France, Germany, Greece, Ireland, Italy, Luxembourg,

	the Netherlands, Portugal, Spain, Sweden, and the United Kingdom
FFS	fee for service
GDP	gross domestic product
HBS	Household Budget Survey
HIV/AIDS	human immunodeficiency virus/acquired immuno-deficiency syndrome
IDU	injecting drug user
LSMS	Living Standards Measurements Survey
MDG	Millennium Development Goal
MIP	Medical Insurance Program (Georgia)
MRI	magnetic resonance imaging
OECD	Organisation for Economic Co-operation and Development
OOP	out of pocket
P4P	pay for performance
PHC	primary health care
RRS	Roma Regional Survey
SHI	social health insurance
TB	tuberculosis
VSL	value of statistical life
WHO	World Health Organization

Overview

If you ask policy makers or technocrats about their country's health system, they will probably start to talk about budgets, hospitals, doctors, drugs, and so on. Ask people on the street, and they are more likely to begin with their personal experience—or that of a parent, friend, or neighbor. They may tell a positive story—of a successful reform or of an illness cured. But it is perhaps just as likely that they will express some frustration—about the costs, the quality, or the complexity. These conversations could take place anywhere in the world, of course. Health is a difficult sector, and it matters to people in a way that few others do. But it is perhaps even more common for unhappiness with the health system to be part of conversations taking place in the countries of Europe and Central Asia (ECA).

This report is about how to improve health system outcomes in countries in the ECA region. Long-term historical trends indicate substantial room for improvement, especially when ECA's health outcomes are compared to those of the EU-15. Instead of catching up with their Western neighbors, many countries in ECA have been falling behind. In addition, over the past decade or more, key outcomes in health financing have not converged with those of the EU-15. The need for accelerated progress is therefore clear.

Achieving better outcomes would also help governments respond to popular demand—that is, for the policy maker to answer to the person on the street—since health is a high priority for populations across the region. This sentiment is likely to become even stronger over time, since living long, healthy lives is an aspiration that tends to grow in importance as countries become richer and basic needs are met. As a result, health sector challenges are here to stay for policy makers throughout ECA.

This report, which explores the development challenge facing health sectors in ECA, identifies three key agendas for achieving more rapid convergence with the world's best-performing health systems:

- The first is the health agenda, in which the main imperative is to strengthen public health and primary-care interventions to help achieve the "cardiovascular revolution" that has taken place in the West in recent decades.

- The second is the financing agenda, in which growing demand for medical care must be satisfied without imposing an undue burden on households, by achieving better financial protection, or on government budgets, by ensuring a more efficient use of resources.

- The third agenda relates to broader institutional arrangements. Here, a few key reform ingredients are identified, each of which is common to most advanced health systems but lacking in many ECA countries.

A common theme in each of these three agendas is the emphasis on improving outcomes, or "getting better."

A Development Challenge

Fifty years ago, the countries of Europe and Central Asia were faring quite well in matters of health. Significant progress had been made in addressing maternal and child health and infectious disease, more than in most other regions of the world. Life expectancy in ECA was just 5 years less than in Western Europe but 10 years more than in Latin America and 20 years more than in East Asia and the Middle East. The region's health outcomes therefore far surpassed those in most other low- and middle-income countries around the globe.

Today, the picture is different. While health outcomes in the region are not far from the global average for the region's income level, the long-term trend has not been good. The life expectancy gap

FIGURE 0.1

Since 1960, Life Expectancy Gains in ECA Have Been the Lowest in the World

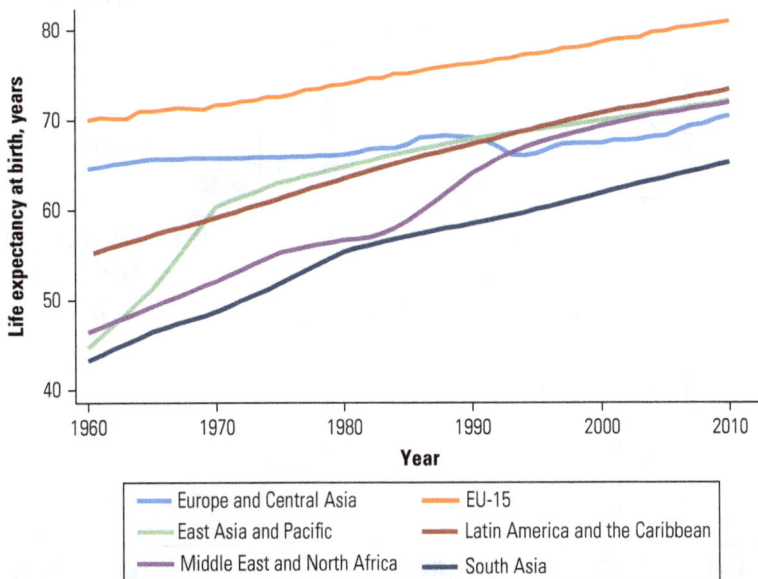

Source: World Development Indicators (database).
Note: Figure shows life expectancy by world region. ECA = Europe and Central Asia.

between ECA and the EU-15 has doubled to about 10 years, and the other middle-income regions have all overtaken ECA (figure O.1). Surveys of global health have noted the tremendous gains in health worldwide over the past half-century, with two major exceptions: Sub-Saharan Africa, due to the HIV/AIDS epidemic, and Eastern Europe (Cutler, Deaton, and Lleras-Muney 2006). The slow progress of ECA's health outcomes is thus of global significance.

The story of ECA's long-term health trends is not uniform (figure O.2). Some countries have performed very well. Turkey is the best example, having added nearly a quarter-century to its life expectancy since 1960, in line with other high-performing middle-income countries. The former Yugoslav republics have also achieved steady health progress over most of this period. Meanwhile, the Baltic nations, Central Europe, and the larger former Soviet republics all experienced almost no improvement in health outcomes between 1970 and 1990. But since then, their trends have diverged. Central Europe has made steady progress, while the former Soviet republics experienced severe declines early in the transition period, from which the Baltics have recovered, while Belarus, the Russian Federation, and Ukraine have not. Central Asia and

FIGURE 0.2

Significant Variation in ECA's Health Trends across Countries and over Time

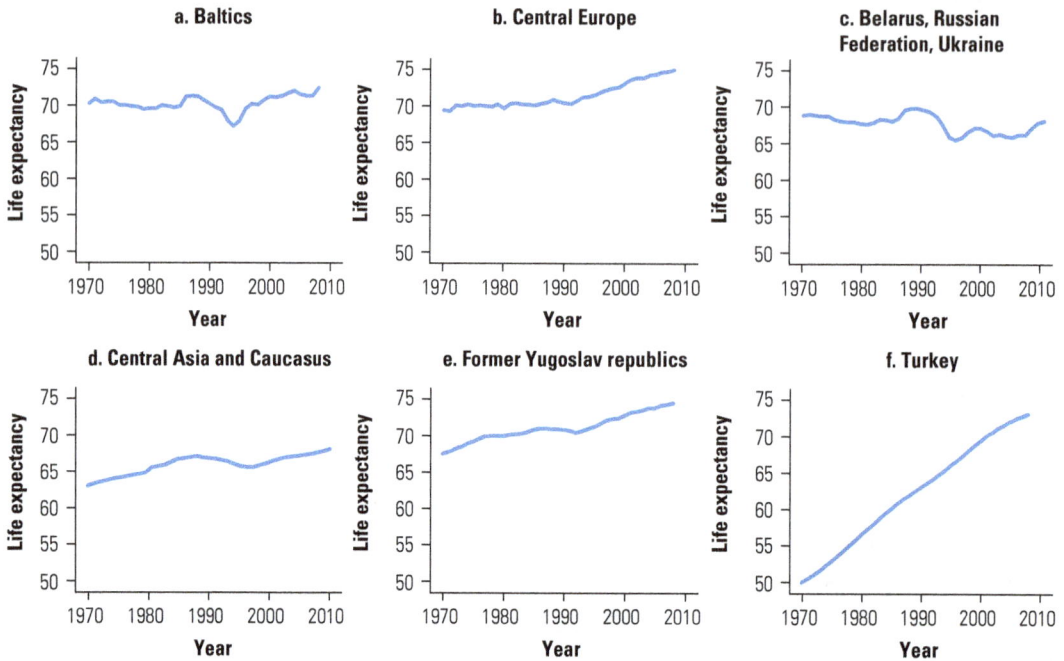

Source: World Development Indicators (database).
Note: Figure panels show life expectancy at birth. ECA = Europe and Central Asia.

the Caucasus did better before 1990 than they have since. Very recently, trends have started to improve in a larger number of countries, but full parity with the EU-15 is still a long way off.

The regional trend also defies simple explanations. Slow progress is not just the product of a difficult period of transition from command to market economies, since the flat trend of health outcomes was apparent well before 1990. Nor does the trend apply only to men, as the life expectancy gain among women since the 1960s has only been about one year higher. And ECA's health challenges are not limited to just one or two large countries, since many countries across the region have struggled to make progress.

The divergence in health indicators between Eastern and Western Europe has come about despite recent progress with convergence in income levels. Although since the mid-1990s the ECA region has enjoyed faster growth in gross domestic product (GDP) than the EU-15, that growth has not translated into more rapid gains in life expectancy. That finding is in line with the global finding that growth does not automatically lead to better health (Deaton 2007). Instead, gains tend to arise from the wider application of health-improving knowledge and technology, particularly in personal behavior and medical care. Concerted public action can play a pivotal role in accelerating this process: it does not happen automatically as a result of higher incomes.

These long-term trends in ECA matter because health is valued so highly. There are many ways to advocate for the policy importance of the health sector. Better health has been justified on the grounds that it is a basic human right, central to development and a key determinant of happiness. The economic approach to valuing health emphasizes the "willingness to pay." Both research and common sense suggest that people are willing to give up a lot of other consumption to improve their odds of living long, healthy lives. In ECA, survey respondents in six countries were about evenly divided when asked to choose, hypothetically, whether they would prefer to live in a country with a European health system or in one with European living standards. It is also true that better health—especially during early childhood—can raise income levels, but this effect is less important than the large, direct contribution of health to overall well-being.

The concept of a high "value of life" reinforces the message that ECA's historical performance with regard to health improvement has been relatively weak by global standards. A body of research that aims to combine health and wealth into a single metric suggests that health gains can be as important as income gains in their contribution to welfare improvement worldwide (Becker, Philipson, and Soares 2005). But in ECA, the contribution of health to welfare (referred to here as "full income"), and therefore to development in the broadest sense, has been very modest (figure O.3). Overcoming this legacy is therefore a key development challenge for the region.

As further evidence of its importance to ECA's development agenda, health is a top priority for populations across the region. According to survey evidence, the health sector consistently ranks as the first priority for additional government spending in about three-quarters of the countries in the region, including among men and women, old and young, rich and poor (figure O.4). The same is true in much of Western Europe as well. Of course, population preferences are not the only consideration in allocation of government budgets, but they should nonetheless be an important voice in those deliberations.

For the foreseeable future, health is likely to remain a key policy challenge for ECA. As countries grow richer and basic needs are met, the importance of health in household preferences becomes even greater. Living longer, healthier lives is preferred to

FIGURE 0.3

Health Has Contributed Very Little to ECA's Development in the Past 50 Years

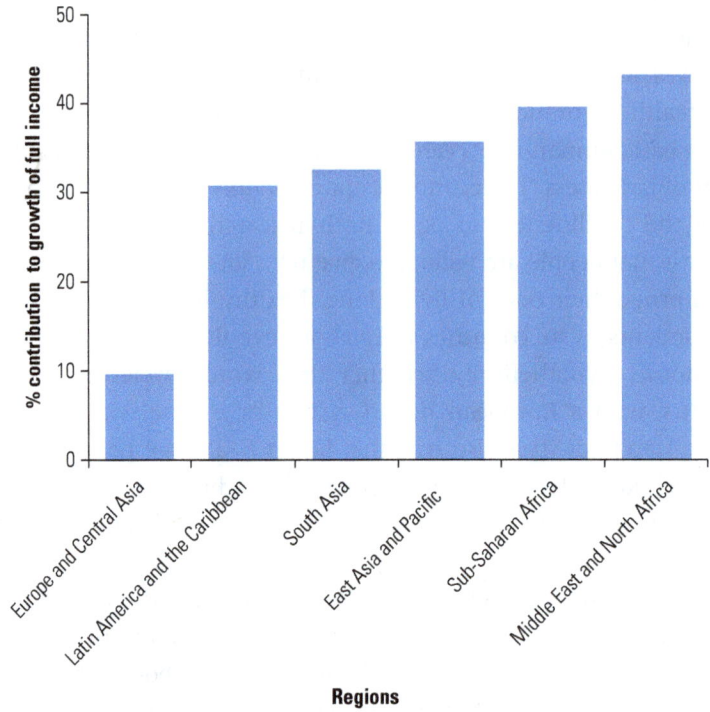

Source: Calculations based on Becker, Philipson, and Soares 2005.
Note: Figure shows the contribution of health to the growth of full income, 1960–2008. ECA = Europe and Central Asia.

FIGURE 0.4

Health Is a Top Priority for Populations across the Region

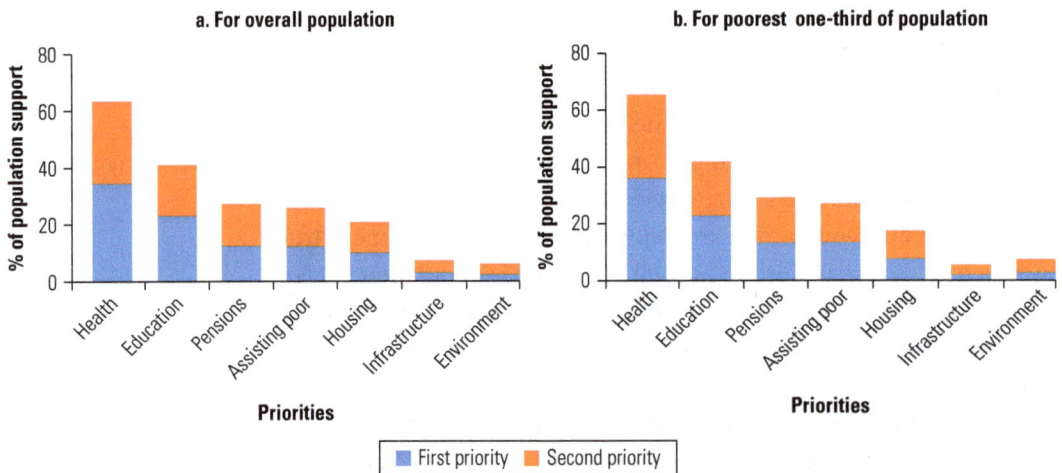

Source: EBRD 2010.
Note: Figure shows the top two priorities for government investment among survey respondents in Europe and Central Asia.

compressing more consumption into a fixed life span. Through surveys, people have typically indicated higher expectations for a government role in health than in other social sectors, such as employment or pensions. By implication, people do not want to be left alone to navigate complex medical care and insurance markets in search of a product that may be life saving or bank breaking—or both, or neither. In brief, the health sector can be expected to take on more prominence in the political agenda of countries across ECA in the years to come.

A road map to the report links the development challenge described here to the three key agendas discussed below (figure O.5). The development challenge corresponds to the ultimate policy objective of improving welfare, of which health (and thus the health agenda) is a major determinant. But people have many other spending priorities that matter for their well-being, too, and thus equally important is the issue of how to pay for better health without imposing undue burden on households or government. This is where the financing agenda fits in. Together, the health and financing agendas embrace three commonly identified policy objectives for health systems: improving population health outcomes, the financial protection of households that seek medical care, and the efficiency of government health spending. Finally, a cross-cutting institutional agenda affects performance across the board.

FIGURE O.5
A Road Map to the Report

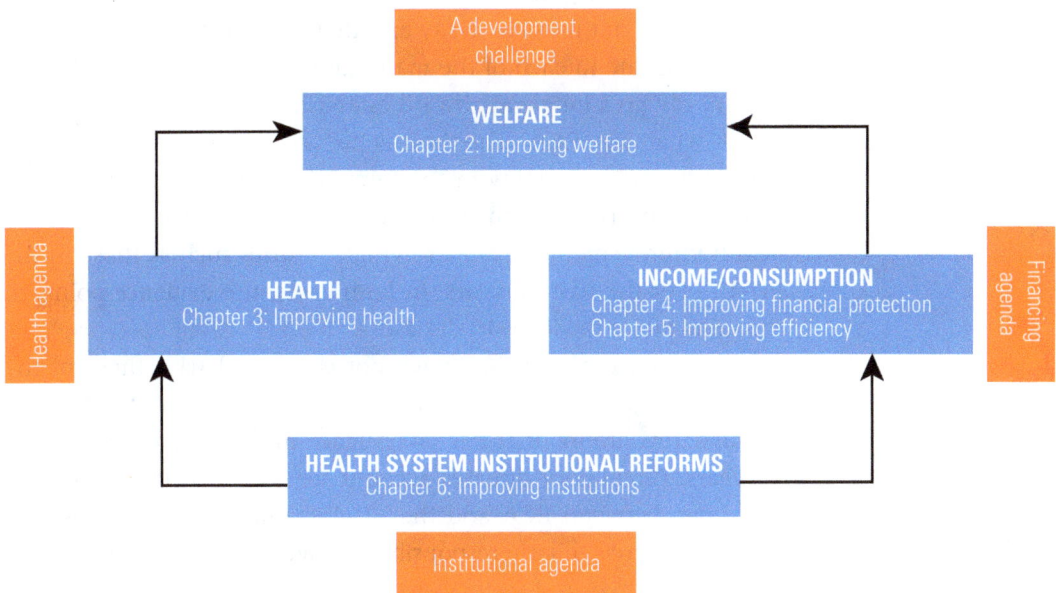

The report brings new evidence to bear on each of these major agendas. A household survey, which was implemented in six countries with a focus on health-related behaviors and utilization of medical care, yielded results that can be compared to existing data sources for all European Union (EU) member states. A quality-of-care survey was undertaken in five countries to assess how providers respond to hypothetical patient "vignettes." Existing household surveys in 11 countries were used to analyze the burden of out-of-pocket spending for health. Last, a questionnaire on the institutional characteristics of health systems was deployed across all ECA countries to systematically assess the health reform agenda across the region. Some cross-cutting themes common to these data collection efforts include benchmarking ECA against the EU-15, balancing an overview of health systems as a whole with a focus on specific diseases, and emphasizing key outcomes or "results" relevant to each of the three agendas.

The Health Agenda: Achieving a Cardiovascular Revolution

Identifying a health policy agenda for ECA should begin with an understanding of why its performance has lagged behind that of other regions. There are many determinants of individual and population health: a list would have to include genes, early childhood conditions, nutrition, knowledge about the factors that affect health, educational level, personal behaviors, the environment, socioeconomic status, and medical care. Each is likely to be relevant for ECA at least to some degree.

While it is not possible to say exactly how much of a population's ill health is due to each of the many underlying causes, two lines of inquiry can go a long way toward establishing a preliminary diagnosis of what ails ECA. The first is to account for the proximate determinants of mortality in the form of common measures of disease burden. The second is to look at the historical evidence on health improvements in longer-living countries such as those in the EU-15 over the past 50 years. In both cases, the evidence points to the same major cause: heart disease.

Health outcomes in ECA have not converged with those of the EU-15 in large part because the region has yet to achieve the "cardiovascular revolution" that has taken place in the West over the past 50 years. Circulatory diseases account for over half the life expectancy gap between ECA and the EU-15, and better cardiovascular outcomes were similarly responsible for over half the health gains in the EU-15 in recent decades (figure O.6). Perhaps more than in any

FIGURE O.6

Cardiovascular Disease Is the Main Source of the Life Expectancy Gap between ECA and the EU-15

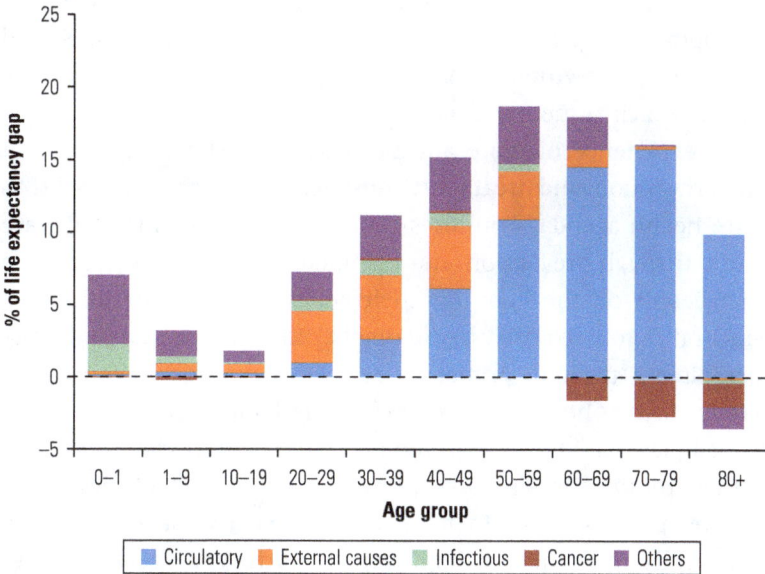

Source: Canudas-Romo 2011.
Note: ECA = Europe and Central Asia.

other field, this is where the miracle of modern medicine has been most evident. In 1950, little could be done to help a patient with heart disease, and knowledge of its causes was very incomplete. Today, much more is known, and a wide range of drugs and technologies is available to help address it. The overwhelming importance of a single disease group, albeit a complex one, should send a clear signal about ECA's lagging health outcomes and represents an obvious target for policy action.

In addition to cardiovascular disease, two other factors behind the life expectancy gap also stand out. The first is neonatal mortality (that is, death in the first 28 days of life), which accounts for the majority of deaths before age one. Improvements on this front, in no small measure due to new medical technologies, have also been a major reason for increased life expectancy in the EU-15. The second is external causes, mainly due to alcohol-related road traffic injuries, which are responsible for an extraordinary and unnecessary loss of life concentrated among the working-age male population in a relatively small number of countries in the region.

The report's emphasis on these factors is not intended to promote more vertical programming but rather to view the health convergence challenge through the lens of a few key conditions and then draw lessons for health systems more broadly. The systemic reforms that can help strengthen these interventions will also contribute to the reduction of other causes of ill health. Other important priorities include an unfinished agenda related to the Millennium Development Goals (especially those related to HIV/AIDS and tuberculosis), the growing challenge of cancer, and major sources of morbidity such as mental health.

The experience of more advanced health systems suggests that both prevention and treatment must play a central role in ECA's future health agenda. Countries cannot entirely avoid their disease burden through prevention, nor can medical care be fully relied on to let people off the hook for their behaviors. More specifically, a reduction in tobacco use, the treatment of risk factors for cardiovascular disease through primary care, better management of acute episodes such as heart attack and stroke, and improved neonatal care have all played a huge role in the health gains in the West in recent decades. Yet there are important shortcomings in each of these areas in many parts of ECA. In brief, the factors that have figured so prominently in the health improvements achieved elsewhere offer important insights in helping identify priorities in ECA today.

The starting point for reducing cardiovascular disease mortality is to address its major risk factors in the general population before people need medical care. Among the most important are tobacco and alcohol use. Men in ECA smoke more than their counterparts in almost any other region and significantly more than in the EU-15. Alcohol use—and more specifically, binge drinking—is also a major problem in some countries. In general, awareness of the health risks associated with tobacco and alcohol use is strong, typically even more so than in Western Europe. A lack of knowledge of the health consequences of risky behaviors does not appear to be a major underlying reason for excessive smoking and drinking in ECA.

While tobacco use is more prevalent, smokers in ECA are also more likely to report that they are trying to quit than those in the EU-15, and they usually cite health concerns as a major reason. Nevertheless, they appear to be less successful at quitting, as reflected in the much higher ratios of smokers to ex-smokers in the population (figure O.7). The large numbers of smokers who are trying to quit, in addition to the significant share of the population that complains of second-hand smoke, provide a strong rationale for government intervention.

In many ECA countries, the anti-tobacco policy environment is less supportive than in the EU-15. The most effective tobacco

FIGURE 0.7

Fewer Smokers Are Quitting in ECA

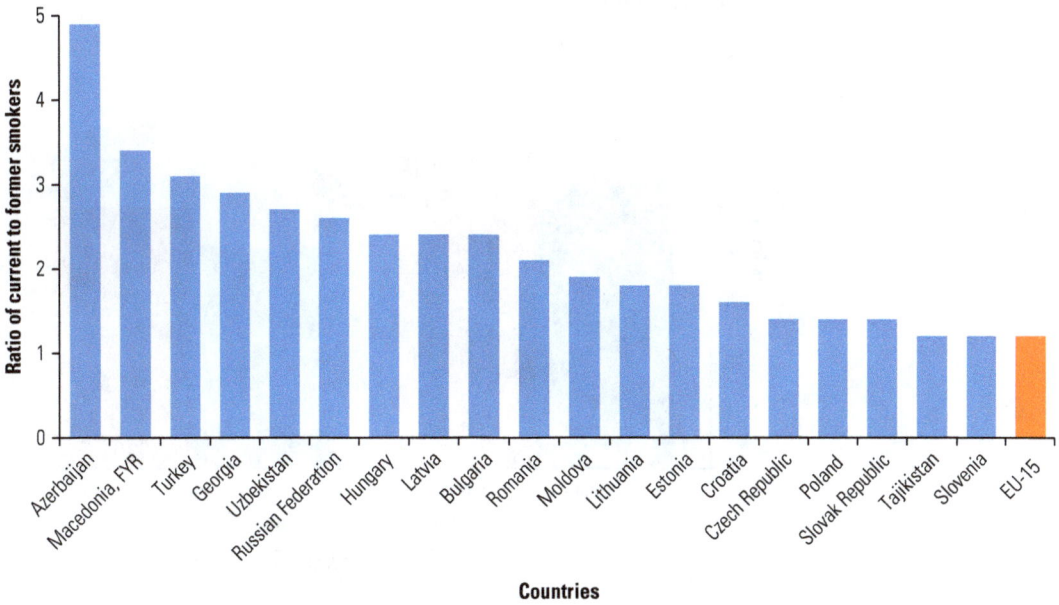

Sources: European Commission 2010; World Bank 2012a.
Note: The figure shows the ratio of current to former smokers. ECA = Europe and Central Asia.

control policy is to increase cigarette taxes, for which strong evidence indicates a significant impact in the form of reduced consumption. But in many cases, tax rates remain quite low. All EU countries have cigarette taxes that exceed 75 percent of retail prices, and most Balkan countries fall just short of that level. Cigarette taxes in most countries in the Commonwealth of Independent States (CIS) are well below 50 percent. The responsiveness of cigarette consumption to price is even higher among youth, and thus tobacco taxation can play a key role in deterring uptake in the first place. Another area in which ECA's anti-tobacco policies lag behind the EU-15 is with respect to smoking bans in public places such as restaurants and workplaces. But there are exceptions. Turkey represents a recent example from within the region of ambitious anti-tobacco reforms being undertaken in a relatively short period of time.

Across the region, there is widespread support for public health measures such as higher taxation and public smoking bans to help address tobacco and alcohol use. But the policies lag behind, suggesting that public opinion is ahead of government action. Women, who smoke and drink significantly less than men yet bear a disproportionate share of the consequences, are even more strongly in favor of

FIGURE O.8

Widespread Support for Anti-tobacco Measures, Especially among Women

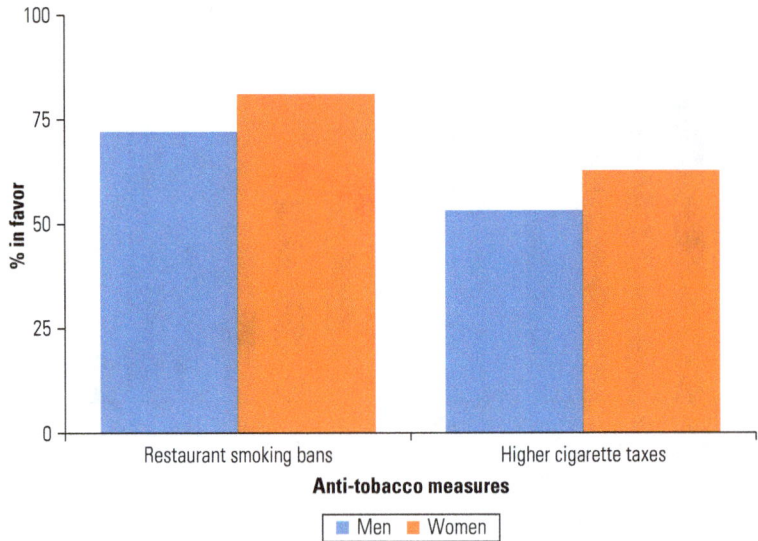

Sources: European Commission 2007, 2010; World Bank 2012a.

stronger anti-tobacco and anti-alcohol policies (figure O.8). The experience of the EU-15 suggests that these reforms will eventually happen and will be popular: the question is not if, but when. Leadership will play a key role in moving the public health agenda forward, not only in the area of tobacco and alcohol, but also with respect to multisectoral challenges related to food regulation, road traffic injuries, and others.

While population-based interventions can play a key role in preventing the emergence of cardiovascular disease, inevitably there will be individuals with risk factors who come into contact with the medical care system, many of whom can be successfully treated through primary care. But cardiovascular risk factors are often not being properly managed in outpatient settings across the region.

Survey respondents in ECA report as many heart checkups and blood pressure measurements as in the EU-15, but after that the results chain appears to break down. High blood pressure is the most important risk factor for premature mortality in ECA, but only about 10 percent of those with the condition in many ECA countries have it under control, compared to over 50 percent in some advanced health systems (figure O.9). Populations are also less likely to be tested for high cholesterol, another major risk factor. The adult population of the EU-15 is almost three times as likely as those in the CIS region to have had a cholesterol test in the past year.

FIGURE O.9

High Blood Pressure Is Not Being Treated and Controlled

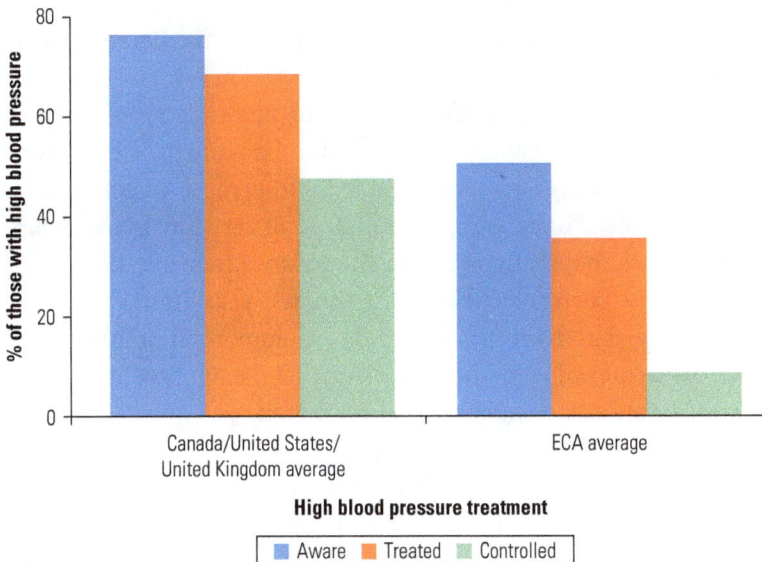

Source: World Bank 2012a.
Note: ECA = Europe and Central Asia.

Various policy measures can help improve the management of these risk factors through primary care. First and foremost, outpatient drug benefit packages to help treat these conditions can be strengthened. In many countries, this is perhaps the most important missing element from today's health benefit packages. The drugs are cheap, and thus the budgetary implications should not be major. While the low costs may be taken as evidence that patients should be able to afford to pay for the drugs themselves, some evidence also suggests that even low copayments for pharmaceuticals can result in nonadherence and can lead to even higher downstream systemwide costs due to more hospitalization episodes.

In the broader system, risk factors should also be more widely measured, monitored, and possibly used as a basis for reimbursement to incentivize physicians through "pay for performance" schemes. Addressing financial considerations, whether on the demand or on the supply side, will not alone solve low treatment and adherence rates. But financial considerations nonetheless represent an important piece of the puzzle. Disease management programs can also help, as can a broader set of institutional reforms to primary care, as discussed below.

Between public health legislation and managing risk factors through primary care, there are major cardiovascular health gains available at very low cost. A big part of the life expectancy gap—probably at least two-thirds and perhaps more—can be addressed through these lower levels of care. As a result, closing the gap does not need to be expensive. The majority of potential health improvements will not involve hospitals; yet these absorb undue attention and resources.

More generally, while people in ECA may visit the doctor as much as those in the EU-15, meaningful service provision to address chronic disease is often lacking. This is true of a wide range of health care provision, from cancer screening to the treatment of depression. For example, cancer screening rates for the most treatable forms (breast, cervical, colon, and prostate) are still very low in many parts of ECA, while populations in the EU-15 are often five times more likely to have been screened during the past year. In brief, many of the services that have proven to be so important in the health advances achieved elsewhere are not yet being provided on an adequate scale across much of the ECA region.

Last, while the emphasis should be on efforts to prevent illness and manage risk factors, health systems must also aim to achieve a high quality of care in the treatment of chronic and acute episodes of illness. One aspect of the quality of care is "structural," referring to inputs such as material resources and staffing, as well as how services are organized. Evidence from five ECA countries surveyed indicates that there are shortcomings in these areas, with respect not only to how well facilities are equipped but also to their management practices. For example, it was found that a large share of hospitals do not have a dedicated committee to oversee quality of care, they do not use checklists for supervision and inventory control purposes, and they do not carry out routine audits of the medical register or in case of a death. Taking steps to address these gaps would help move the quality-of-care agenda forward.

A second, more important aspect of the quality of care relates to "clinical process," or the interaction between the health worker and the patient. Global evidence suggests that this is more closely associated with health outcomes than the presence of structural inputs. To measure this dimension of the quality of care in ECA, a survey was undertaken in five countries that used clinical "vignettes"—an approach that simulates an actual patient encounter—to assess how providers would treat hypothetical patients. These included acute episodes of major cardiovascular and neonatal events such as heart attack, birth asphyxia, and neonatal pneumonia. The findings highlight major problems with quality of care. On average, less than 60 percent of the maximum score was achieved across all services. For example, less than two-thirds of doctors surveyed across five countries correctly diagnosed a heart attack when faced with a hypothetical patient with all the clinical signs of

FIGURE 0.10

The Quality of Key Health Care Services Can Be Improved

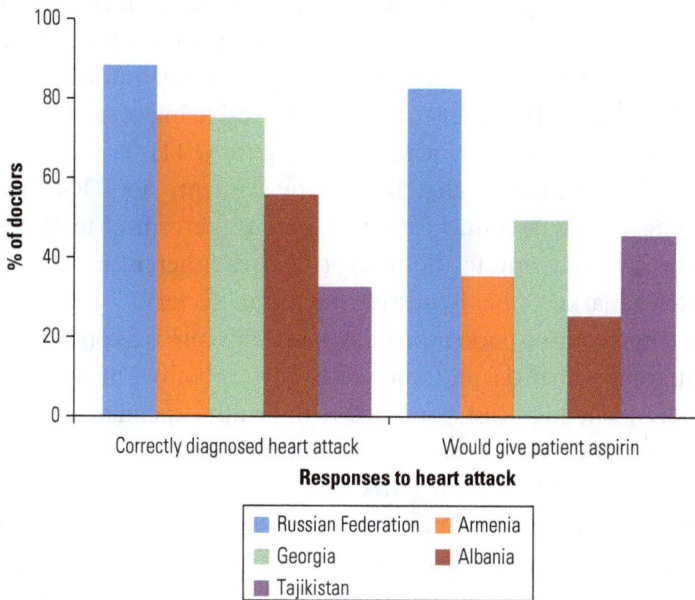

Source: World Bank 2013.
Note: Figure shows provider responses to clinical vignette of heart attack. Results for the Russian Federation are from
Kirov oblast.

one, and less than half said they would give the patient aspirin, a
crucial step in helping prevent further blood clotting (figure O.10).
A range of measures can help address shortcomings in the clinical
process. Many of these involve better performance measurement that
can be linked to payment, professional recognition, and peer review.

The Financing Agenda: A Safety Net for All—While Cutting the Fat

Making progress on the health agenda raises the equally challenging
question of how to pay for it. This is the focus of the financing
agenda. Everywhere the demand for health care is substantial: each
year about 1 to 2 percent of any population will be born or die, with
associated costs; people get sick, the body breaks down, and accidents
happen. Most countries in ECA and around the world spend between
5 and 10 percent of GDP in total on health (public and private), or
somewhat more in richer, older countries and somewhat less in
poorer, younger nations. The global experience has also been that
health spending steadily increases over time. With a large and growing share of income spent on health, the policy challenge is to ensure
that this money buys better outcomes.

The financing agenda must satisfy this growing demand for health care without imposing an undue burden on households or the government budget. Both in ECA and globally, health financing is drawn largely from either household out-of-pocket (OOP) sources or from the government budget (that is, through tax revenues, including mandatory social health insurance). The relative importance of these two sources varies widely across ECA (figure O.11). Private, voluntary health insurance—that is, nongovernment, non-OOP health spending—rarely accounts for more than 10 percent of total health spending, largely due to the market failures inherent in individual insurance markets (that is, outside the formal sector).

Too much out-of-pocket spending for health care is a concern when it undermines financial protection or equity (or both). The uncertainty and potentially high cost associated with health expenditures—we do not know when we might fall sick, and how much it will cost if we do—impose sizable spending risk on households. As a result, OOP expenditures for health may be "catastrophic"—that is, exceeding some significant threshold (for example, 10 percent) of total household expenditures—or "impoverishing," if they push some households below the poverty line. OOP expenditures can also pose an important barrier to access to health care, and the resulting inequalities in utilization between rich and poor should be a concern to policy makers.

FIGURE O.11

The Balance between Out-of-Pocket Spending and Government Budgets Varies Widely

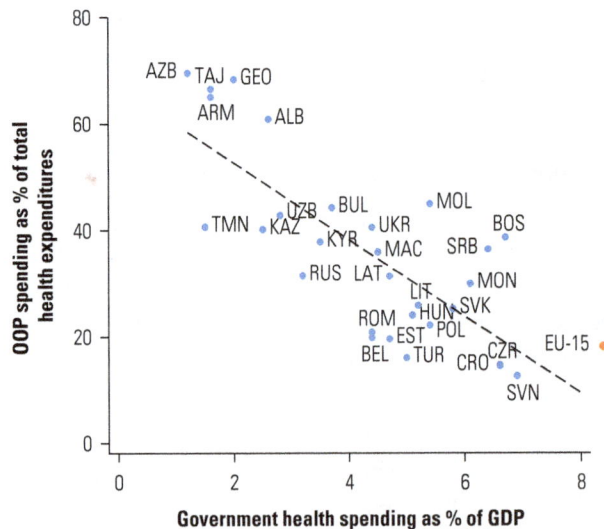

Source: WHO 2012.
Note: GDP = gross domestic product; OOP = out-of-pocket spending.

Very few countries in ECA have significantly reduced their reliance on out-of-pocket payments, a key indicator of financial protection, since 1997. In fact, nearly twice as many countries in the region have had an increase instead of a decline. The gap between ECA and the EU-15 on this front remains essentially where it was 15 years ago and thus represents another challenge for health system convergence.

Inadequate financial protection due to high OOP payments remains a problem in about half the ECA region. Households in these countries spend a larger and less predictable share of their total resources on health than their counterparts in the EU-15—in several cases more than twice as much on average (figure O.12). A large share of this spending is on drugs, and much of it is catastrophic. Household survey data from across the region show that the more heavily a country relies on OOP payments for health financing, the more common these catastrophic episodes become, the greater the inequality is in utilization of care across socioeconomic groups, and the more people fall into poverty as a result of their medical bills (figure O.13).

The objective should not be to lower OOP spending to zero, but relying on this source for 40–70 percent of total heath financing, as in many ECA countries, can create an important gap in safety nets. Catastrophic health care episodes represent well over half of total

FIGURE O.12

Substantial Out-of-Pocket Payments for Health in ECA, Especially for Drugs

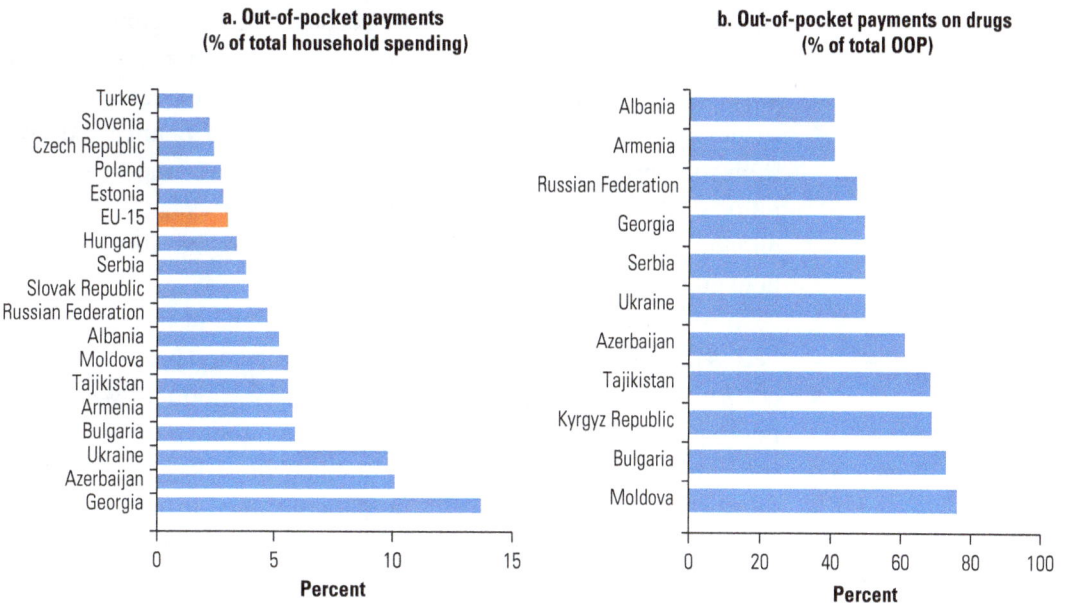

Sources: OECD 2011; Ali and Smith 2012.
Note: ECA = Europe and Central Asia; OOP = out-of-pocket.

FIGURE 0.13

A Greater Reliance on Out-of-Pocket Payments Undermines Financial Protection and Leads to Inequality in Use

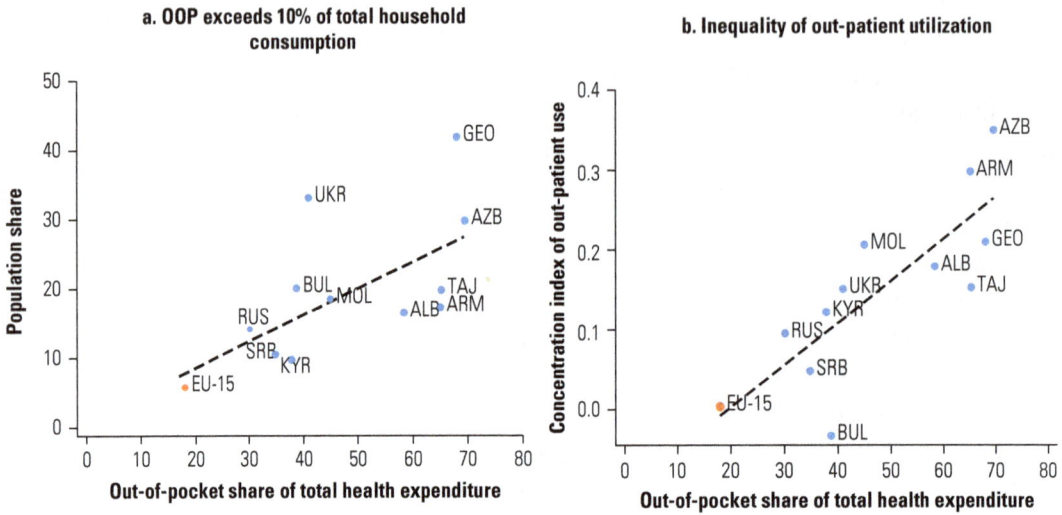

a. OOP exceeds 10% of total household consumption

b. Inequality of out-patient utilization

Source: Ali and Smith 2012.
Note: GDP = gross domestic product; OOP = out of pocket.

OOP spending in many ECA countries. And while traditional theory has emphasized the problem of overutilization due to moral hazard, newer theories from behavioral economics put a greater emphasis on underuse, especially of highly cost-effective preventive services. This underuse can also have financial consequences for the system as a whole. Once the various reasons to achieve lower OOP spending are summed up, theory and evidence would suggest that less than 25 percent of total health financing drawn from this source is a reasonable policy objective. In the EU-15, the ratio is 18 percent. Careful design of benefit packages—including difficult decisions about which services cannot be afforded—can help guide progress on this front.

In some countries—especially those with small health budgets—a necessary step for strengthening financial protection is through more government health spending. How to spend additional resources to improve financial protection will vary from country to country. In some cases, it will mean expanding the benefit package, especially in the form of better coverage of outpatient drugs. In others, it may require better reimbursement of underpaid providers to help deter informal payments. Still elsewhere there may be specific populations, such as those working in the informal sector, that are not adequately covered by existing programs. In some countries of Central and

Eastern Europe, access to health care among the Roma population could be strengthened.

Special effort should be made to ensure that improvements in financial protection and access to care benefit the poorest first, through targeted health programs. Better-off households typically have more options for obtaining health coverage and are more resilient in the face of unexpected medical bills. But the poor and near-poor are much more vulnerable. Georgia offers a successful example of using a proxy means test to target additional health resources to the poor.

But more government spending is not always necessary and does not automatically translate into improved financial protection outcomes. Rent seeking by health care providers in the form of informal payments and high pharmaceutical price markups are also important causes of weak financial protection in ECA. Achieving better outcomes may therefore require some supply-side measures to address informal payments and high drug spending. In the case of medical staff, this effort may entail stronger accountability mechanisms and patient empowerment. Armenia's recent success with its maternity voucher reform offers a good example in this regard. For drugs, there is a need for clear treatment protocols, drug lists, generic promotion, and, potentially, price regulation. Together, these can help address overprescription, overconsumption, and overspending.

Concerns about the burden of excessive spending apply equally to government health budgets, which are often wasteful and pose a threat to fiscal sustainability. The size of health budgets varies widely across the region, from just over 1 percent to nearly 7 percent of GDP, compared to an average of 8 percent in the EU-15 (figure O.14). In fact, the level of government health spending in ECA has not risen as fast as in the EU-15 or in other middle-income regions, including East Asia and Latin America, since the late 1990s, either as a share of GDP or as a share of the total government budget. But amid growing population demands and a tight fiscal environment, the efficiency of spending remains a major concern in the region. Every country offers scope for better use of existing resources.

Excess hospital infrastructure is a key source of waste. In the CIS region, there are nearly twice as many hospitals per person as in the EU-15. That excess results in high fixed costs, unnecessarily long admissions, and hospital beds that are occupied for the wrong reasons: for example, in some ECA countries people are up to 10 times more likely to be hospitalized for hypertension than in the EU-15, a condition that should be controlled at lower levels of care. Often the major constraint to reducing hospital capacity is political will, but

FIGURE 0.14

Government Health Budgets in ECA Cover a Wide Range but Are Smaller than in the EU-15

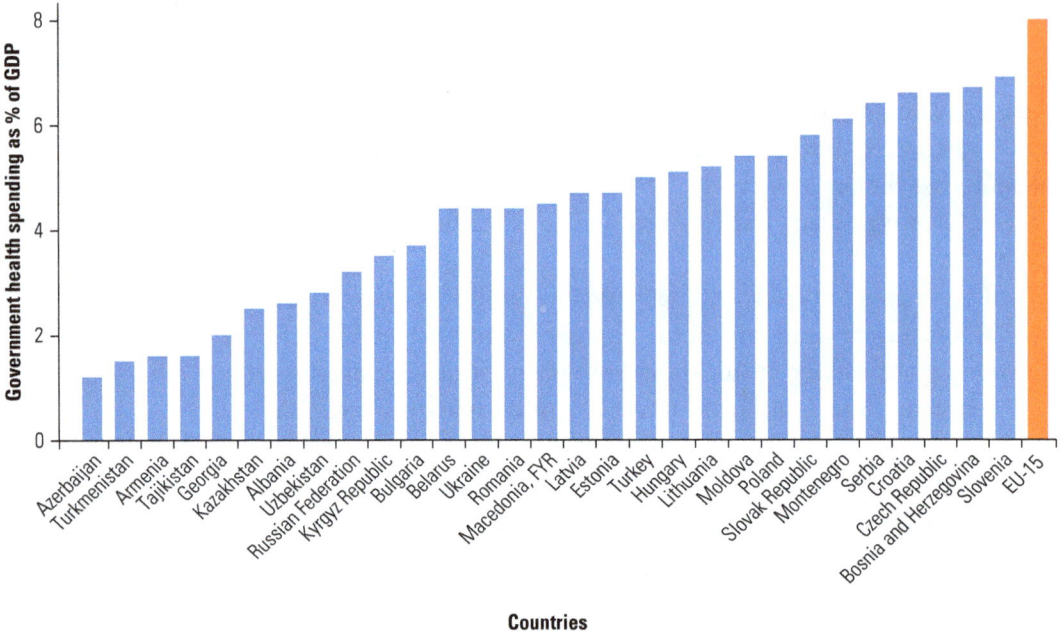

Countries

Source: WHO 2012.
Note: ECA = Europe and Central Asia; GDP = gross domestic product.

some countries in the region have successfully made these reforms. Hospital downsizing should be accompanied by service delivery innovations, such as one-day surgeries and more attention to primary care. Ultimately, it is in the interest of the health system and patients alike for a population to spend less rather than more time in hospital.

Across ECA, pharmaceuticals are an additional major driver of excess costs. The burden of drug spending is not a problem limited to OOP spending, as governments across the region struggle to contain the pressure that these exert on their budgets. Smarter procurement of drugs will play a key role in improving results, including through more sophisticated contracting approaches to help achieve lower prices. Croatia offers a strong example from the region of how this can be done.

More generally, there are few silver bullets for the efficiency agenda. Some commonly cited proposals to improve efficiency have important caveats. For example, while prevention programs are very important as a way to promote better health, when spread across an entire population, they are not automatically cheaper than treatment. Similarly, as noted, more patient cost sharing might result in cutbacks of unnecessary care, but there is also evidence that people will cut back on very cost-effective care, potentially leading to higher downstream costs. Finally, simple prescriptions for more competition among insurers and providers do not necessarily translate into better value for money.

A major challenge is that while health systems often have a large amount of waste, at their best they also provide some life-saving care. The imperative is to find a way to cut one without cutting the other. Health systems simultaneously overprovide and underprovide various services. For example, X-rays are administered more often in most ECA countries than in the EU-15, while the opposite is true of flu vaccinations among the elderly—a highly cost-effective (and even cost-saving) intervention that should be offered far more widely. Blunt, cross-cutting policy instruments may not adequately distinguish between the two: trimming the fat will usually require a scalpel, not a sword.

A significant and sometimes overlooked part of the agenda is not about pursuing major systemic reforms but rather about under-standing "micro" variation in outputs and outcomes across different providers and services. For example, some doctors refer more patients to higher levels of care, order more diagnostic procedures, or prescribe more drugs than their colleagues. Similarly, some hospitals have higher readmission rates or higher mortality rates for specific types of care than others. The organizations that pay for services should keep track of these patterns and make use of this information to address the outliers through more active approaches to purchasing care.

Last, while the financing agenda puts the focus on the cost of health spending, passing judgment on any policy or program requires some effort to consider the benefits, too. Cutting government health spending or stopping its growth is easy—for example, hard budget caps could be imposed on all facilities beyond which no reimburse-ment would be made—but improving welfare is an altogether more difficult task. Ultimately, health expenditure pressures in middle- and high-income countries are due to the growing importance that people place on living a long, healthy life, once basic needs are met, as highlighted earlier. For this reason, long-term growth in spending on health in the West has, on the whole, been worth it, even in the presence of significant waste, because of the high value attached to health gains achieved through medical advances. In brief, cost containment will not always be the right strategy. The challenge is therefore to ensure that when additional resources are spent, as they almost surely will be, they are translated into improved outcomes instead of more waste.

The Institutional Agenda: Ingredients, Not Recipes

A health system's underlying institutional arrangements affect both the health and the financing agendas. The institutional agenda embraces topics such as how a system is financed, how service delivery is organized, and what regulations are in place. Many reforms have been undertaken in these areas over the past 20 years, but the agenda remains unfinished. The relatively slow convergence of health and financial protection outcomes with the EU-15 may be to some extent attributable to the overall institutional characteristics of ECA's health sectors.

While benchmarking is more straightforward for health outcomes and financial protection, it is more difficult in the case of institutional reform, given that it is not immediately clear what a "developed" health system looks like. For this reason, a systematic review of ECA's health systems, using an approach already implemented across 29 Organisation for Economic Co-operation and Development (OECD) countries, was undertaken as a benchmarking exercise. The objective was to answer two questions. First, to what extent have the institutional characteristics of OECD health systems converged? And second, where this convergence has occurred, to what extent have ECA health systems also evolved toward this common approach? The results highlight the heterogeneity that exists among advanced-country health systems but also some common tendencies.

Based on this exercise, a policy agenda for ECA's health systems is proposed on the grounds that it is possible to identify "ingredients," but not "recipes," for institutional reform of health systems. In other words, it is possible to identify certain common characteristics of countries with strong health systems, but not a fully articulated model (which would require specifying the quantities and sequencing of various measures), because no single recipe exists. This approach borrows from the narrative developed in the context of identifying a policy agenda for achieving economic growth (Commission on Growth and Development 2008), a complex task that arguably has similarities to the health reform agenda.

Five key ingredients are proposed for the agenda to reform the institutions of ECA's health systems. Although not universal among OECD countries, these ingredients are very widespread and are becoming more so. The first three ingredients are all closely tied to the concept of accountability in service provision. The first of these is some degree of activity-based reimbursement, or "payment follows the patient." In primary care, this implies the use of fee-for-service methods, even if only partially in the form of a mixed system with other approaches. It may also take the form of a pay-for-performance scheme. An important complement to activity-based payment is patient choice. In hospitals, activity-based payment commonly takes the form of diagnosis-related groups in OECD countries, and many countries in ECA have started to move in this direction. Other approaches are possible, including methods that combine activity-based reimbursement with other options. The absence of this ingredient would be signified in the primary-care setting by payment of salary alone or a pure capitation model (although this may serve as a useful transition arrangement) and in the hospital setting by line-item budgeting or pure global budgeting. Yet these approaches persist in many ECA health systems.

The second ingredient is provider autonomy, or the extent to which a facility has "decision rights" over the many aspects of producing health care services, including labor and capital inputs, output level and mix, and management processes. In the OECD, provider autonomy is typically achieved in primary care in the form of private solo or group practices, whereas public primary-care provision continues to predominate in the CIS region. In hospitals, public ownership is the norm across all regions. But differences between OECD countries and ECA are particularly apparent in whether hospital managers have complete autonomy for the recruitment of medical staff and other health professionals or if the central or local government decides. Over two-thirds of OECD health systems extend this autonomy, compared to about half of western ECA and only one-quarter of eastern ECA.

Provider payment and autonomy work best hand in hand. Creating payment-based incentives without the decision-making power to act on them is likely to fall short of achieving intended objectives. On this front, primary care in many ECA countries looks to be further from the OECD norm than in the case of hospitals, as figure O.15 illustrates. Only three OECD countries have no element of fee-for-service payment, no patient choice, and limited autonomy in the form of publicly provided primary care, while over half the countries in the eastern part of ECA have this model. Over three-quarters of health systems in the OECD and in the western part of ECA have at least two of these three accountability mechanisms, whereas in the CIS region only two countries fit this category. The pattern of payment and autonomy arrangements for primary care in ECA represent a key potential explanation for the shortcomings in primary-care delivery, including control of the cardiovascular risk factors described earlier. Reforms in this area will be an important step toward improving outcomes.

The third ingredient is the use of information for decision making. Health systems may produce thousands of individual services at hundreds of different facilities on a daily basis, and there is likely

FIGURE O.15

Accountability of Primary Care Is Stronger in OECD Health Systems than in ECA

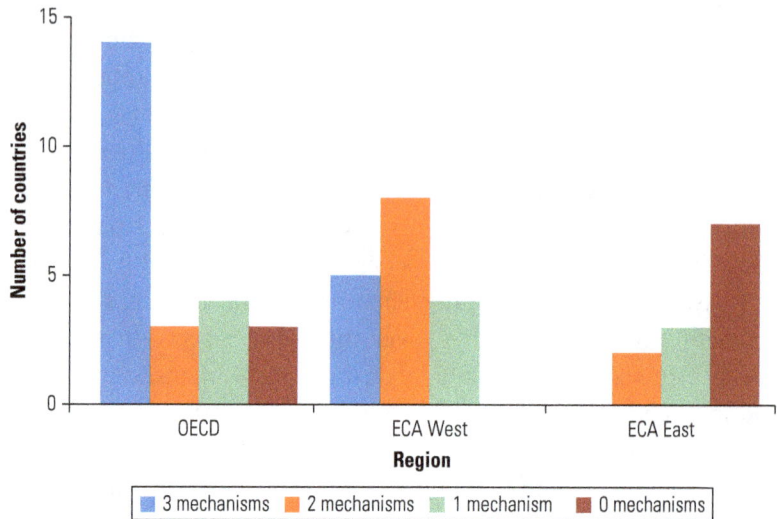

Sources: Paris, Devaux, and Wei 2010; World Bank 2012b.
Note: Figure indicates the number of primary care accountability mechanisms, including activity-based payment, provider choice, and autonomy for primary care. OECD = Organisation for Economic Co-operation and Development; ECA = Europe and Central Asia.

to be significant variation in performance across both these dimensions. The availability of information flows to monitor and act on this variation is important for ongoing system improvement. Figure O.16 illustrates the differences across the OECD and ECA with respect to several examples of health systems' use of information. Each of these can make an important contribution to achieving better quality and efficiency. Individually, these measures are not uniformly used across the OECD, but the tendency is in that direction. In the health systems of eastern ECA, these information tools are almost nonexistent.

The fourth ingredient is adequate risk pooling. Many aspects of health financing—such as how revenues are raised, whether coverage is automatic or compulsory, and whether there is a national health service, a single insurer, or multiple insurers—vary widely across the OECD, offering few clear lessons for others seeking to chart their way forward. But irrespective of these questions, nearly all OECD countries have high levels of risk pooling that are not too fragmented and do not rely on voluntary means. In brief, health financing in the OECD has converged in coverage levels but not in institutional design. Thus, the health-financing policy agenda for ECA is chiefly to expand coverage of people and services through

FIGURE O.16

Health System Capacity to Use Information Is Less Developed in ECA than in the OECD

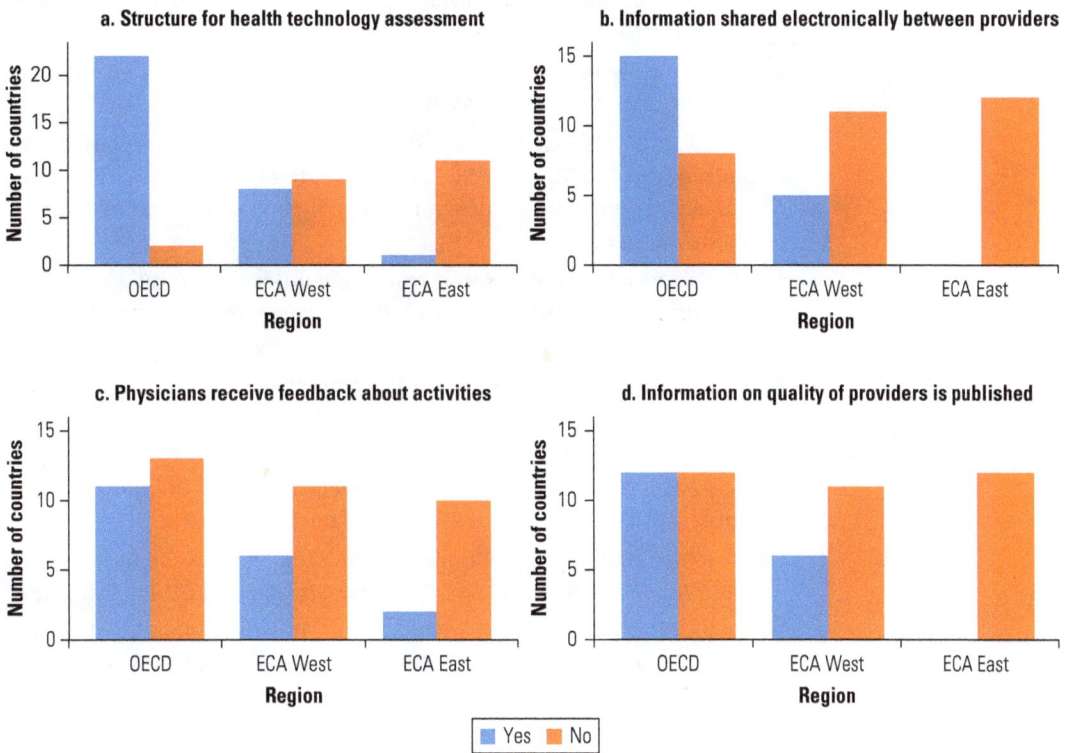

a. Structure for health technology assessment

b. Information shared electronically between providers

c. Physicians receive feedback about activities

d. Information on quality of providers is published

Sources: Paris, Devaux, and Wei 2010; World Bank 2012b.
Note: OECD = Organisation for Economic Co-operation and Development; ECA = Europe and Central Asia.

adequate risk pooling, with more than a single feasible institutional approach available to do so.

The final ingredient in moving the health reform agenda forward is committed, credible leadership. This requirement was also posited as a key policy ingredient in the context of achieving more rapid economic growth. Vested interests will need to be overcome, but there is popular demand for stronger health systems across the region. The difference between being five years ahead of the curve on this policy challenge or five years behind will be a decade of better health system outcomes.

References

Ali, R., and O. Smith. 2012. "Financial Protection and Equity in Europe and Central Asia." Draft. World Bank, Washington, DC.

Becker, G. S., T. J. Philipson, and R. R.Soares. 2005. "The Quantity and Quality of Life and the Evolution of World Inequality." *American Economic Review* 95 (1): 277–291.

Canudas-Romo, V. 2011. "Mortality Decomposition." Background paper for ECA regional health report, World Bank, Washington, DC.

Commission on Growth and Development. 2008. *The Growth Report: Strategies for Sustained Growth and Inclusive Development.* Washington, DC: World Bank.

Cutler, D., A. Deaton, and A. Lleras-Muney. 2006. "The Determinants of Mortality." *Journal of Economic Perspectives* 20 (3): 97–120.

Deaton, A. 2007. "Global Patterns of Income and Health: Facts, Interpretations, and Policies." UNU-WIDER Lecture, September 26, 2006, Princeton University, http://www.princeton.edu/rpds/papers/pdfs/deaton_WIDER_annual-lecture-2006.pdf.

EBRD (European Bank for Reconstruction and Development). 2010. *Life in Transition Survey,* http://www.ebrd.com/pages/research/publications/special/transitionII.shtml.

European Commission. 2007. Eurobarometer 66.2, October–November 2006. TNS Opinion & Social, Brussels. GESIS Data Archive ZA4527, dataset version 1.0.

———. 2010. Eurobarometer 72.3, October 2009. TNS Opinion & Social, Brussels. GESIS Data Archive ZA4977, dataset version 1.0.

OECD (Organisation for Economic Co-operation and Development). 2011. *OECD Health at a Glance 2011: OECD Indicators.* Paris: OECD Publishing.

Paris, V., M. Devaux, and L. Wei. 2010. "Health System Institutional Characteristics: A Survey of 29 OECD Countries." OECD Health Working Paper 50, Organisation for Economic Co-operation and Development, Paris.

World Bank. 2012a. "Findings from a Household Survey on Health in 6 ECA Countries." Draft. World Bank, Washington, DC.

———. 2012b. "Health System Institutional Characteristics in ECA." Draft. World Bank, Washington, DC.

———. 2013. "Findings from a Quality of Care Survey Using Clinical Vignettes in 5 ECA countries." Draft. World Bank, Washington, DC.

World Development Indicators (database). World Bank, Washington, DC, http://data.worldbank.org/data-catalog/world-development-indicators.

World Health Organization. 2012. National Health Accounts database, http://www.who.int/nha/expenditure_database/en.

CHAPTER 1

Getting Better?
In Search of Convergence

Key Messages

- The three major objectives of all health systems are to improve population health outcomes, protect households against the high and uncertain costs of medical care, and ensure the efficiency of government health spending. How to improve these three outcomes is the focus of this report.

- The life expectancy gap between ECA and Western Europe has widened significantly since the 1960s, while other middle-income regions have caught up and overtaken ECA. Some countries are doing better, and very recently there has been an improved trend, but the region has significantly underperformed over many decades.

- Very few countries in ECA have significantly reduced their reliance on out-of-pocket payments—a key indicator of financial protection—since 1997. The gap between ECA and the EU-15 on this front remains essentially as it did 15 years ago. Financial protection remains a problem in about half the countries in ECA.

- Since the late 1990s, the level of government health spending in ECA has not risen as fast as in the EU-15, either as a share of GDP or as a share of the total government budget. Although welcome from a cost containment perspective, this lack of convergence may also be at the expense of other sectoral objectives.

- The objective of this report is to understand the main factors behind the relatively slow long-term convergence of key health sector outcomes between ECA and the EU-15 as described in this chapter and to identify policies to help overcome them.

Fifty years ago, the health systems of Europe and Central Asia (ECA) compared favorably with most others in the world. The challenges of infectious diseases and maternal and child health were being systematically addressed, and outcomes were improving to an extent that far surpassed those in most other low- and middle-income countries around the globe. In addition, people did not have to pay dearly for these benefits. In the West, indicators were slightly better, but the imminent explosion of knowledge and technology that would help revolutionize human health could not have been easily foreseen. In short, ECA was faring quite well in matters of health.

But times have changed. Today, if you ask policy makers or technocrats in ECA about their country's health system, they will probably start to talk about budgets, hospitals, doctors, drugs, and the like. Ask people on the street, and they are more likely to begin with their personal experience—or that of a parent, sibling, friend, or neighbor. You hope to hear a positive story—of a successful reform or of an illness cured. But it is perhaps more likely that you will hear of some frustration—about the costs, the quality, or the complexity. Similar conversations could take place anywhere in the world, of course. Health is a difficult sector, and it matters to people in a way that few others do. But in some important respects, and particularly given the starting point 50 years ago, the view in ECA is justified.

We begin this report by looking at some of the evidence that gives voice to the concerns of both the policy maker and the person on the street. Many of ECA's health systems are no longer faring so well, regardless of whose perspective is taken. But there are some success stories, and those are deserving of attention as well. Some countries are putting the historical legacy behind them and embarking on a healthy future. In this chapter, we begin with a brief overview of health sector trends and then offer a preview of how the report is organized.

Some Successes, but Overall Slow Progress on Key Objectives

The performance of a health sector should be assessed with reference to its major objectives. This report is organized around a view that the three major goals of a health sector are (1) to improve health outcomes (both the level and distribution); (2) to provide financial protection against the potentially high and uncertain costs of ill health; and (3) to ensure that health spending is efficient. These goals also correspond to the first three strategic directions identified in the World Bank's strategy for health, nutrition, and population results (World Bank 2007). This section will briefly survey the landscape in ECA with respect to these three major goals or "results." Each one is also the subject of a chapter later in this report.

A recurring question is whether there is evidence of *convergence* with the 15 member countries of the European Union (EU) prior to 2004 (henceforth, EU-15) with respect to these objectives. While it is not generally expected that ECA would currently have outcomes on a par with its Western counterparts, it is natural to ask whether the gap is being closed. Are these outcomes getting better? As we will see, on average there has been relatively little long-term convergence between ECA and Western Europe on key health sector objectives, albeit with significant country variation. This observation—both the underlying causes and how they can be overcome—is the main motivation and focus of this report.

We begin with health outcomes. The most basic indicator is life expectancy at birth, a simple, widely reported metric of the length of life. Along with gross domestic product (GDP) per capita, it is arguably one of the two most important indicators of a country's level of development, since together they capture (albeit imperfectly) the quantity and quality of life. It will be our benchmark indicator of a country's health outcomes. Of course, other indicators are important, too. Infant, child, and maternal mortality are particularly important to those groups and are at the heart of the Millennium Development Goals health agenda. In addition, mortality-based indicators should be complemented by measures of morbidity (sickness), such as disability-adjusted life years lost.

FIGURE 1.1

On and off the Curve

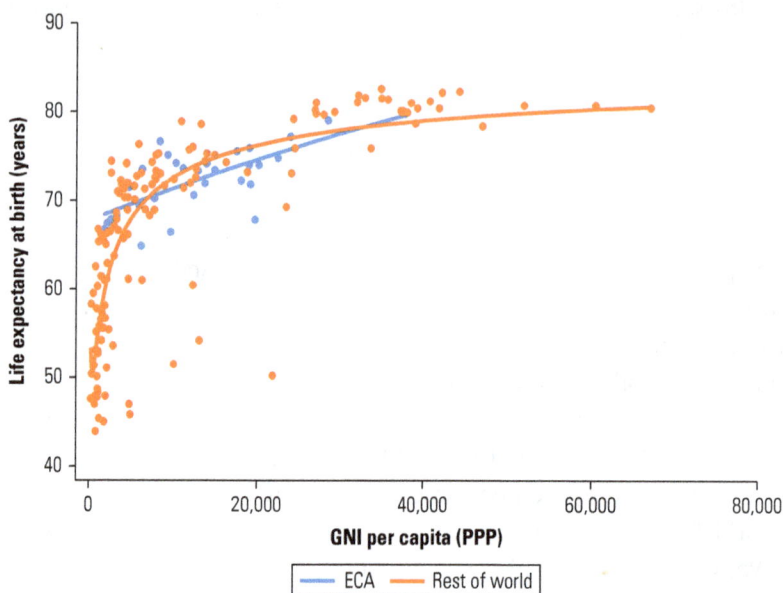

Source: World Development Indicators (database).
Note: Data points indicate years of life expectancy in various countries in ECA and rest of the world. ECA = Europe and Central Asia; GNI = gross national income; PPP = purchasing power parity.

How does ECA's life expectancy measure up against the world? Figure 1.1 shows this comparison sorted by income per capita, also known as the Preston curve (Preston 1975). Many ECA countries are "on the curve," while several others are on the "inside," implying that there are many other countries with either lower income and the same life expectancy or the same income and greater longevity (or a little of both). The farthest ECA country from the curve is the Russian Federation.

While the average life span in most of ECA today is not dramatically worse than global averages, a closer look at long-term historical trends provides a more sobering view of the region's performance (figure 1.2). As suggested from the outset, average life expectancy in ECA in 1960 was almost 65, just five years less than in Western Europe and much higher than in today's other middle-income regions. By 2010, ECA's life expectancy had only recently passed 70, leaving it about a decade behind the EU-15. Several ECA countries have the same life expectancy today as the EU-15 did 50 or more years ago. Meanwhile, three other middle-income regions—East Asia, Latin America, and the Middle East—have all surpassed ECA, with an average life span of close to 73 years. Since 1985, ECA has added barely two years to its life expectancy. Very recently—since

FIGURE 1.2

Since 1960, Life Expectancy Gains in ECA Have Been the Lowest in the World

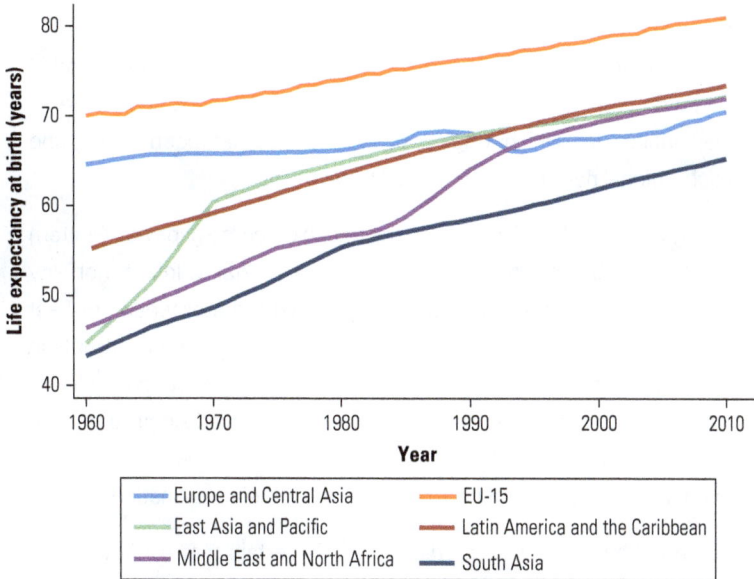

Source: World Development Indicators (database).
Note: Figure shows life expectancy by world region. ECA = Europe and Central Asia.

2007—there has been a slight improvement, but it is too early to conclude that all is well again (Wang et al. 2012).

ECA's long-term record appears even weaker if Turkey is excluded from the regional average, as it represents over 15 percent of the region's population and its life expectancy has risen by a quarter-century, from 48 years to 73, over this time. In fact, there is significant cross-country variation, both over time and space, as discussed in box 1.1.

Certain patterns underlying figure 1.2 are especially worthy of note as they may run counter to common perceptions. First, the stagnation of trends started in the late 1960s, and so it is not simply a side effect of transition. The early 1990s certainly witnessed a deterioration of health outcomes, but evidence suggests that even that is not closely associated with economic hardship, but rather due to other factors (box 1.1). Second, the flat trend is common across both men and women—the longevity gain since 1970 among women has been only 1.1 years higher than among men. Third, the regional trend is not driven entirely by one or two larger countries such as Russia and Ukraine. To varying degrees, there are also laggards among small and

A Brief Historical Tour of Health Trends in ECA: Different Countries, Time Periods, Narratives

The slow progress of life expectancy in ECA, as shown in figure 1.2, masks considerable variation across countries and over time. Broadly speaking, three distinct periods can be identified, but there are also clear outliers for which long-term performance has been strong and steady. A brief overview of subregional narratives is provided here:

- *Catching up, 1950–70.* During this period, ECA narrowed the health outcome gap with Western Europe, much of which was due to big improvements in under-five mortality. Infant mortality was cut in half, a faster rate than in other middle-income regions with the exception of East Asia. This progress was particularly marked in the Soviet Union, where large improvements in nutrition and public health measures to address infectious diseases were responsible for better outcomes. Child height, adult height, and infant mortality all improved significantly during the postwar period in the USSR (Brainerd 2010). The expansion of public health and education programs and improved caloric and nutrient intake are the most likely explanations.

- *Stagnation, 1970–90.* This period has been less studied, but it is certain that cardiovascular disease (CVD) mortality remained stubbornly high up until some improvements in the mid-1980s (Shkolnikov, Mesle, and Vallin 1996). Alcohol consumption had started to increase sharply in the 1960s and 1970s. Meanwhile, CVD mortality began to plummet in the West, thanks largely to improved medical care and a decrease in smoking prevalence (Cutler, Deaton, and Lleras-Muney 2006). Medical technology improvement did not penetrate ECA to a significant extent (figure B1.1.1a).

- *Divergence, 1990–2010.* In the early transition period, mortality rates surged in several former Soviet republics. This has been the subject of a large research literature (Brainerd and Cutler 2005; Shkolnikov et al. 2004; Stillman 2006). The evidence points to a number of conclusions: (1) alcohol played a key role, especially related to cardiovascular disease and injuries (homicide, suicide, and road traffic injuries), but also past mortality patterns resumed, following the repeal of the successful Gorbachev-era policies (Bhattacharya, Gathmann, and Miller, forthcoming); (2) a deterioration of law and order was associated with a greater frequency of reckless driving and violence; and (3) much of the mortality trend is not fully explained, but it is believed that changes in diet, health care provision, and general economic activity did *not* have a large impact on mortality rates. Meanwhile, a rapid improvement was seen in Central Europe (the Czech Republic, Hungary, Poland, and the Slovak Republic) in the 1990s (figure B1.1.1a). This has been attributed to both dietary changes and improved access to medical technologies (Brainerd 2012).

- *Outliers.* Several exceptions to the main trend are also noteworthy. Turkey's experience more closely reflects that of other middle-income countries, and indeed it has rapidly caught up

continued

BOX 1.1 *continued*

with its comparators around the world (Baris, Mollahaliloglu, and Aydin 2011). Perhaps a more puzzling exception has been the western Balkans, where life expectancy has improved at a fairly steady rate (with the exception of a period from the mid-1970s until 1990) over the past 50 years. Potential hypotheses include the mitigating role of diet (Gjonca 2004) and a larger emphasis on primary care than in the Soviet Union (Davis 2010) (figure B1.1.1b).

FIGURE B1.1.1

Significant Variation in Life Expectancy Trends across Countries and over Time, 1970–2010

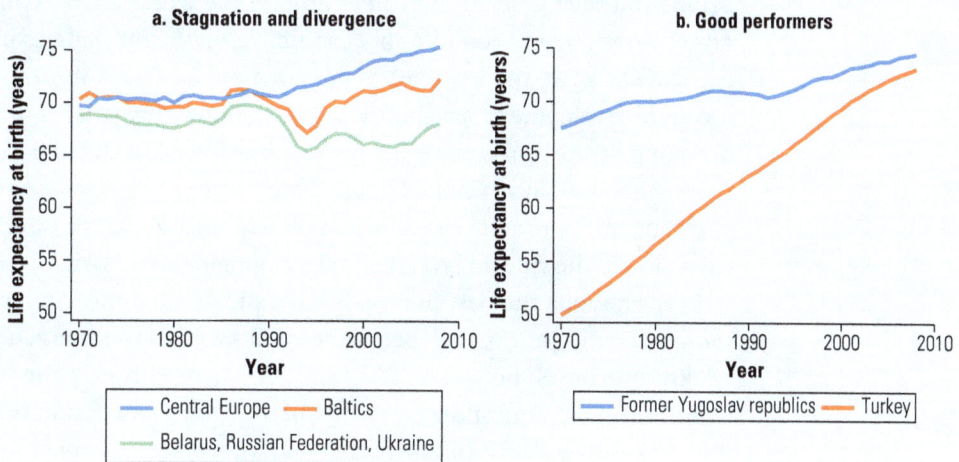

a. Stagnation and divergence

b. Good performers

Legend: Central Europe — Baltics — Belarus, Russian Federation, Ukraine — Former Yugoslav republics — Turkey

Source: World Development Indicators (database).

large countries from the Baltics to the Caucasus and from Central Asia to southeast Europe. Finally, while alcohol plays an important role in excess mortality in some countries, it is by no means the only culprit—there are many other causal factors, as discussed in chapter 3.

The catch-up of other middle-income countries is mostly due to their later success in addressing infant and child mortality, which have a disproportionate impact on life expectancy. The contrast with ECA is therefore partly the consequence of ECA's early successes in addressing these issues in the 1950s. But it is also true that available evidence on adult mortality suggests that ECA has underperformed on this measure since 1970 vis-à-vis others (Rajaratnam et al. 2010).

However, the divergence from Western Europe is particularly striking. The gap in life expectancy has doubled, from about 5 to 10 years, since 1960. By contrast, the dominant global demographic trend in the 20th century was *convergence* of life expectancy across countries. In the late 20th century, this trend began to falter, because of two major exceptions: the HIV/AIDS pandemic in Sub-Saharan Africa, and the health crisis in Eastern Europe (Moser, Shkolnikov, and Leon 2005). ECA's stagnant health outcomes are thus of global significance.

Diverging health trends are also in contrast to ECA's converging income per capita with Western Europe since the early 1990s (World Bank 2012). On the surface, this may seem surprising. If people are growing richer, why is health not improving? But a closer review of the evidence suggests this mechanism is generally quite weak. There is little evidence that economic growth is a significant causal factor behind improving health outcomes around the world: there is almost no relationship between rates of economic growth and changes in life expectancy over the past 50 years (Deaton 2007). But from the broader development perspective, it is noteworthy that Europe's diverging health and converging income levels are just the opposite of the global norm, in which health outcomes have converged (as above), while income per capita has diverged (Pritchett 1997). Thus, ECA is an exception to the rule on both major development indicators.

In sum, while the past five years have shown an improving trend, the long-term pattern has been one of slow or no convergence of health outcomes between ECA and Western Europe. The most important policy question raised by the foregoing discussion is how this long-term pattern can be permanently reversed. As noted, this is a major motivating issue for this report and will be addressed in depth in chapter 3.

As we turn to the second major objective of a health system, long-term financial protection, we see that trends across countries in ECA reveal a few success stories, but overall very little convergence. The uncertainty and potentially high cost associated with health expenditures—we often do not know when we will become sick and how much it will cost if we do—make them amenable to prepayment and risk-pooling arrangements. Over time, successful policy initiatives can help countries shift their health financing arrangements away from direct out-of-pocket (OOP) payments by households. There are different ways to measure financial protection. Here we focus on the share of total health expenditures accounted for by OOP payments. As discussed in chapter 4, reliance on OOP payments is strongly cor-related with other measures such as the incidence of impoverishing and catastrophic OOP spending, as well as inequality in utilization.

Since 1997 (the earliest year with reliable data), the reliance on out-of-pocket payments has increased on average across ECA, but with significant cross-country variation (see figure 1.3). Twice as

FIGURE 1.3

More Backward Steps than Forward Steps on Financial Protection

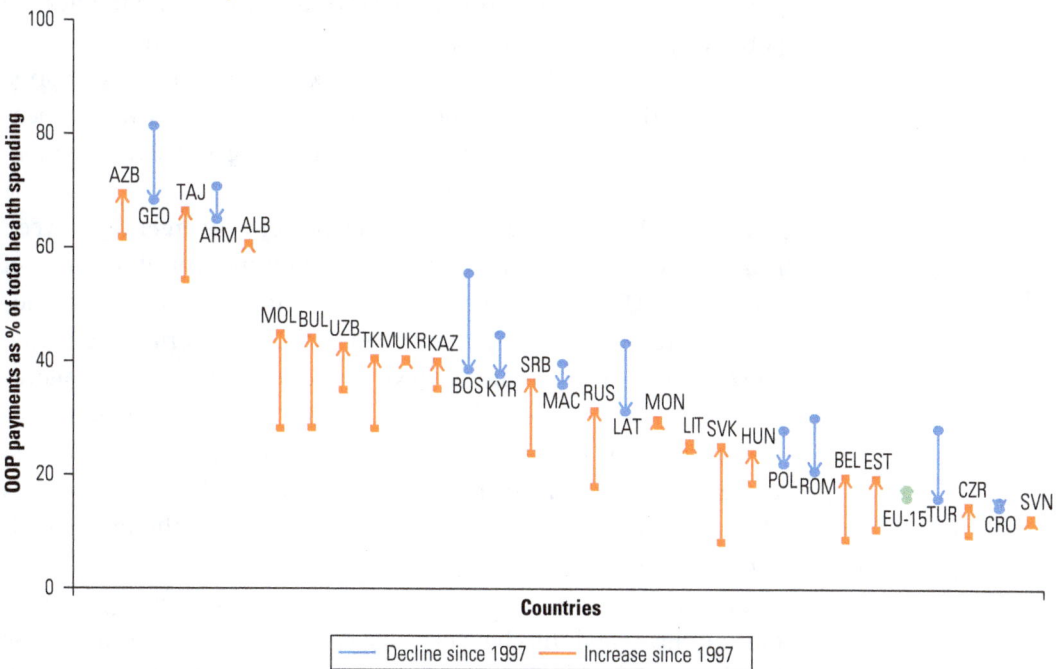

Source: WHO 2012.
Note: Figure shows changes in share of out-of-pocket payments, 1997–2010. OOP = out of pocket.

many countries have witnessed a rise in OOP spending as compared to a fall, and twice as many have had an increase of at least 10 percentage points compared to those with an equivalent fall. Bosnia and Herzegovina, Latvia, Romania, and Turkey show the most favorable trends. The sharpest increases in OOP reliance are observed in Bulgaria, Moldova, Russia, Serbia, and the Slovak Republic. In other countries, such as Albania, Tajikistan, and the three countries of the south Caucasus, OOP spending remains persistently high.

Of course, the objective of financial protection is not to lower out-of-pocket payments to zero. But it is noteworthy that OOP payments account for a steady 15–20 percent of total health expenditure in the EU-15, a number broadly consistent with old and new theories on the economic rationale of health financing. About half of ECA is over twice that level. All told, financial protection remains an important issue—either because of persistently high levels or a sharply deteriorating trend—in a little under half of ECA countries. In brief, these are the places where convergence remains elusive.

The other side of the health financing equation is the efficiency of the government health budget, the third major health system objective. The experience of advanced nations—where health spending has typically increased at a rate of nearly two percentage points faster than GDP growth over several decades—underlines the potential pressures that health spending can place on the fiscal environment. Ensuring that this is money well spent is thus a key priority. But measuring efficiency is not straightforward. For now, we focus on trends in overall government health spending and leave the more detailed discussion for chapter 5.

Once again, there is not much evidence of convergence between ECA and Western Europe (figure 1.4). Only five countries, four of them new EU member states, have increased the share of their budget allocated to health by more than the EU-15 during the period 1997–2010. Fifteen countries have reduced their budgetary allocation to health over this period. When health spending is expressed as a share of GDP, only two countries—Bosnia and Herzegovina and Turkey—have seen a larger increase than the EU-15. Over two-thirds of ECA has not seen this ratio increase at even half the rate experienced in Western Europe.

Up until the recent crisis, there was steady economic growth in much of ECA, and thus budgets have risen in real terms. But because health spending usually grows faster than GDP per capita in countries

FIGURE 1.4

A Mostly Positive Picture on Cost Containment, 1997–2010

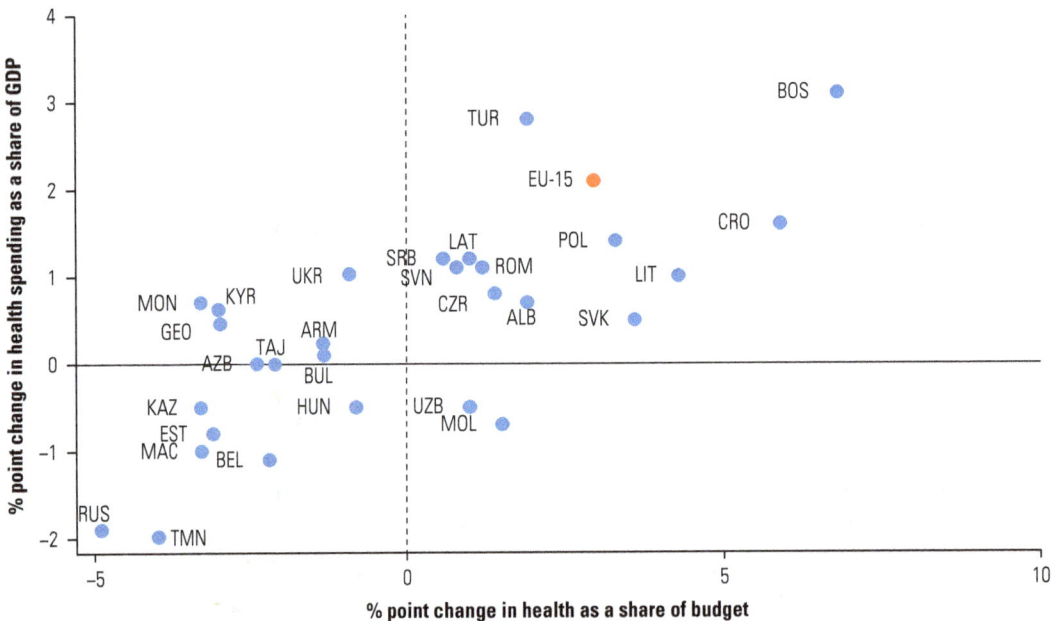

Source: WHO 2012.
Note: Figure shows changes in government spending on health. GDP = gross domestic product.

around the world, including in rapidly growing East Asia, ECA's performance on this front at a time of robust growth is notable.

But unlike in the case of the other objectives, it is not clear whether the lack of convergence of health spending should be interpreted in a positive or a negative light. While successful cost containment may be welcome in a narrow sense, spending trends may also be holding back the achievement of the two earlier objectives. In any event, the efficiency of government health spending is a concern that is unlikely to go away. We will explore these issues in greater depth throughout this report, and especially in chapter 5.

In sum, there has been relatively little convergence between ECA and Western Europe with regard to key health sector indicators. It is not a uniformly negative story—in some countries and on some objectives there is positive news as well. But overall, the data point to an important policy agenda going forward. How to make progress on that agenda will be the focus of the report.

Last, a focus on trends and objectives that may appeal to the technocrat should not come at the expense of some attention to the population's perspective noted at the outset. Achieving more rapid convergence also means a higher degree of satisfaction with the health sector for populations across ECA on the basis of their personal or family experience. Not surprisingly, there is a gap in this regard. For example, the Gallup World Poll (Gallup 2012) asked households whether "in this country, do you have confidence in health care or medical systems, or not?" In the EU-15, 74 percent of respondents said yes, whereas across the ECA region—in both the countries in the Commonwealth of Independent States (CIS) and the new EU member states—the average was close to 50 percent. Interestingly, in the EU-15, respondents had more confidence in their health care systems than in their national governments. In the CIS, it was the opposite: people had more confidence in their governments than in their health systems. While opinion polls do not offer the final word on policy issues, they do represent an important voice. We will revisit some of this evidence in chapter 2.

A Guide to the Report: Objective, Road Map, and Cross-Cutting Themes

The objective of this report is to understand the main factors behind the slow convergence of key health sector indicators between ECA and the EU-15 described above and to identify policies to help overcome them. The main audience is policy makers in ECA, especially those in ministries of finance and health, as well as broader policy circles engaged in health sector issues in these countries and with international agencies. The reality of ECA's long-term health sector struggles is not new, but as the years go by, its policy urgency only increases.

Figure 1.5 provides a road map to help organize the way forward. In the simplest of terms, the health sector is about better health and how to pay for it. That is, it is about improving health in a way that does not impose excessive financial burden on either households (financial protection) or on government budgets (efficiency). Both better health and money for other priorities are important to people: they are both direct contributors to overall welfare. Underlying the road map are the elements of a conceptual framework familiar to economists—a welfare maximization problem.

Since improving welfare is the overall objective of policy applied to any sector, the road map begins there and will explore the contribution of both health and income to that goal (chapter 2). We then proceed to focus on the slow pace of convergence in four respects. We start with health and its determinants and discuss what can be done to improve outcomes (chapter 3). Next we look at the other side: how to ensure that the potentially costly and uncertain financial burden that may be associated with ill health does not impose undue suffering on households (chapter 4), which have other spending priorities as well. This is followed by a similar discussion about mitigating the efficiency losses that the health sector may inflict on government budgets (chapter 5). They too have many other spending priorities. Finally, the "health" and "money" issues are unified once again in a broader discussion of the institutional policy agenda

FIGURE 1.5
A Road Map to the Report

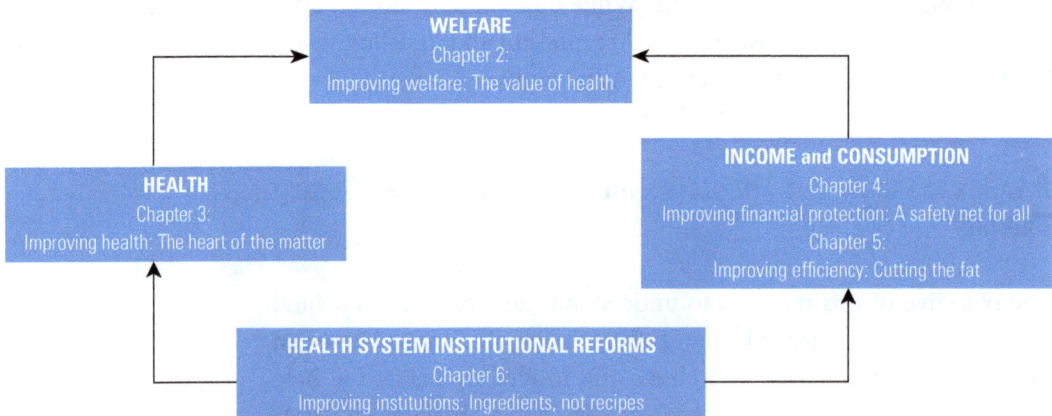

(chapter 6). Here we will address the "macro issues" that tend to dominate discussions of the reform agenda—how to organize service delivery, how to pay providers, how to raise and pool resources for health, and so on. Specifically, we look at the extent to which a lack of institutional convergence helps explain the slow progress of key outcomes. An important theme here is accountability. In keeping with the title of this report, *Getting Better*, each chapter is about improving a specific priority or result.

At this stage, it is also worth highlighting some cross-cutting themes that will recur throughout the report. These are as follows: (1) a focus on outcomes; (2) benchmarking against the EU-15; (3) a balance between a "systems" and a "disease" focus; and (4) a data-driven approach. Each is discussed briefly here:

- *Focusing on outcomes.* The road map has already hinted at a results focus in the report. We begin with what we want to ultimately achieve, an improvement in overall welfare, and work backward from there. Less abstract than welfare, the major results are better health outcomes, more financial protection, and greater efficiency: hence, the three major chapters devoted to these topics. A renewed focus on results is also currently a prominent theme in development policy more broadly.

- *Benchmarking against the EU-15.* The issue of convergence has already been highlighted. Throughout the report, key indicators for ECA countries will be reported alongside the same metric for the EU-15 wherever possible. While Western European health systems are not perfect, they are among the best performing in the world on many of the goals we care about and thus provide a strong indication of what can be achieved. Besides offering a benchmark of what is possible, their historical experience also provides valuable insights into some of the trends that may lie ahead for ECA. Other regions offer useful lessons and benchmarks as well and will be cited at times too, but we emphasize the EU-15 experience as the natural lodestone for an ECA region in which half or more of the countries are currently members of the EU or aspire to membership, while for many of the others, it is a major trading partner and travel destination.

- *Balancing a "systems" and "disease" focus.* Understanding and overcoming the challenges in health sectors require that attention be given both to "systems" issues (such as financing, organization, and the like) and to specific diseases. A business analyst will study a large corporation with reference to its overall revenues, costs, and profits, as well as its individual product lines; an economist will analyze a country's performance in terms of overall growth as well as specific sectors and industries. And so it is with a health sector. Both systems and disease-specific metrics provide meaningful benchmarks for international comparisons, for monitoring the performance of individual hospitals and clinics, and for judging whether a particular reform is working. Our disease focus is mainly on cardiovascular disease and neonatal conditions, as these account for such a large proportion of the disease burden, as discussed in chapter 3. But many others will be cited too. The purpose is not to promote more vertical programming, but rather to identify health system challenges through a disease-specific lens. The efficiency agenda highlighted in chapter 5 can also benefit from some disease-specific analysis.

- *Data driven.* We rely on a wide range of data sources for the analysis in the report and, where appropriate, comment on measurement issues and empirical gaps. A good data flow is essential for many aspects of health sector reform, and strengthening routine information systems should accompany almost any policy initiative undertaken. Box 1.2 provides more background on some of the data used in the report.

BOX 1.2

A Note on Data Sources

This report draws on a range of data sources. Basic cross-country indicators such as life expectancy and infant mortality rates are drawn from the World Bank's World Development Indicators database. These tend to be slightly different from both the World Health Organization and UN Population Division estimates. In some countries, particularly in Central Asia and the Caucasus, all three tend to be lower than country-reported life expectancy, due to considerable uncertainty about the numbers. This difference reflects a combination of factors, including incomplete death registration and different definitions of neonatal mortality (Aleshina and Redmond 2005; Duthe et al. 2010). In some cases, these issues are compounded by uncertainty about the denominator—that is, the overall population is not known within a margin up to 10 percent.

Other data sources include a tailored household survey conducted in 1,000–1,500 households in each of six countries: Azerbaijan, Georgia, Moldova, Russia, Tajikistan, and Uzbekistan. This borrowed heavily from other survey questionnaires, particularly the Euro-barometer studies that included health-related special modules between 2005 and 2009. This approach allowed for cross-country comparisons of many indicators that are not commonly available. The topical focus of this survey was health-related behaviors and utilization of medical care among adult populations.

continued

BOX 1.2 *continued*

TABLE B.1.2.1
Main Survey Data Sources

Survey, year of fieldwork, and implementing agency	Countries
World Bank ECA regional health report household surveys; 2011; World Bank	Azerbaijan, Georgia, Moldova, Russian Federation, Tajikistan, and Uzbekistan
Euro-Barometer special health modules; 2005–09; European Commission	EU-27; Croatia; Macedonia, FYR; and Turkey
World Bank ECA regional health report quality of care surveys; 2012; World Bank	Albania, Armenia, Georgia, Russian Federation, and Tajikistan
ECA household surveys for financial protection and equity analysis; 2007–11; National Household Budget Surveys and World Bank Living Standard Measurement Surveys	Albania, Armenia, Azerbaijan, Bulgaria, Georgia, Kyrgyz Republic, Moldova, Russian Federation, Serbia, Tajikistan, and Ukraine
OECD health system institutional characteristics survey; 2009; OECD	All OECD countries except the United States
ECA regional health report institutional characteristics survey; 2011; World Bank and World Health Organization European Observatory	All ECA countries except those in the OECD

Note: OECD = Organisation for Economic Co-operation and Development; ECA = Europe and Central Asia.

A quality-of-care survey was also carried out in five countries (Albania, Armenia, Georgia, Russia, and Tajikistan), using the approach of clinical practice vignettes. These provide doctors (and nurses) with hypothetical patients and explore how medical professionals would approach patient history, examination, diagnosis, and treatment. This process was accompanied by facility surveys to better understand the physical environment in which medical professionals operate.

The chapter on financial protection draws heavily on Living Standard Measurement Surveys and Household Budget Surveys across the region, a valuable source of data on household utilization and expenditures for health. These findings can be readily disaggregated by socioeconomic status.

Finally, the OECD health system institutional characteristics questionnaire was also administered in 25 ECA countries to systematically take stock of the reform agenda in the region. The report also draws on the substantial literature on health sector issues in the ECA region and, where appropriate, the West.

Finally, the ECA region is diverse, and although the wide variation in country performance is highlighted throughout the report, some statements that are made about the region as a whole for convenience may risk overgeneralization. In broad terms, health system performance has been stronger in the western part of ECA than in countries farther east, and this distinction is emphasized particularly in chapter 6. But there are enough exceptions to the rule—for example, relatively slow progress in health outcomes in the Baltics or weak financial protection in some parts of the Balkans—that it was decided not to identify and formalize specific country groupings for use throughout the report.

References

Aleshina, N., and G. Redmond. 2005. "How High Is Infant Mortality in Central and Eastern Europe and the Commonwealth of Independent States?" *Population Studies* 59 (1): 39–54.

Baris, E., S. Mollahaliloglu, and S. Aydin. 2011. "Health Care in Turkey: From Laggard to Leader." *British Medical Journal* 342: c7456.

Bhattacharya, J., C. Gathmann, and G. Miller. Forthcoming. "The Gorbachev Anti-Alcohol Campaign and Russia's Mortality Crisis." *American Economic Journal: Applied Economics.*

Brainerd, E. 2010. "Reassessing the Standard of Living in the Soviet Union: An Analysis Using Archival and Anthropometric Data." *Journal of Economic History* 70 (1): 83–117.

———. 2012. "The Demographic Transformation of Post-Socialist Countries: Causes, Consequences, and Questions." In *Economies in Transition: The Long-Run View*, edited by Gerard Roland, 57–83. Basingstoke, Hampshire, U.K.: Palgrave Macmillan.

Brainerd, E., and D. Cutler. 2005. "Autopsy of an Empire: Understanding Mortality in Russia and the Former Soviet Union." *Journal of Economic Perspectives* 19 (1): 107–30.

Cutler, D., A. Deaton, and A. Lleras-Muney. 2006. "The Determinants of Mortality." *Journal of Economic Perspectives* 20 (3): 97–120.

Davis, C. 2010. "Understanding the Legacy: Health Financing Systems in the USSR and Central and Eastern Europe prior to Transition." In *Implementing Health Financing Reform: Lessons from Countries in Transition*, edited by J. Kutzin, C. Cashin, and M. Jakab. Geneva: World Health Organization.

Deaton, A. 2007. "Global Patterns of Income and Health: Facts, Interpretations, and Policies." UNU-WIDER Lecture, September 26, 2006, Princeton University. http://www.princeton.edu/rpds/papers/pdfs/deaton_WIDER_annual-lecture-2006.pdf.

Duthe, G., I. Badurashvili, K. Kuyumjyan, F. Mesle, and J. Vallin. 2010. "Mortality in the Caucasus: An Attempt to Re-Estimate Recent Mortality Trends in Armenia and Georgia." *Demographic Research* 22 (23): 691–732.

Gallup World Poll (database). 2012. Gallup Inc. https://worldview.gallup .com/default.aspx.

Gjonca, A. 2004. "Explaining Regional Differences in Mortality in the Balkans: A First Look at the Evidence from Aggregate Data." *EuroHealth* 10 (3/4): 10–14.

Moser, K., V. Shkolnikov, and D. A. Leon. 2005. "World Mortality 1950–2000: Divergence Replaces Convergence from the Late 1980s." *Bulletin of the World Health Organization* 83 (3): 202–09.

Preston, Samuel H. 1975. "The Changing Relation between Mortality and Level of Economic Development." *Population Studies* 29 (2): 231–48.

Pritchett, L. 1997. "Divergence, Big Time." *Journal of Economic Perspectives* 11 (3): 3–17.

Rajaratnam, J., Jake R. Marcus, Alison Levin-Rector, Andrew N. Chalupka, Haidong Wang, Laura Dwyer, Megan Costa, Alan D. Lopez, and Christopher J. L. Murray. 2010. "Worldwide Mortality in Men and Women Aged 15–59 Years from 1970 to 2010: A Systematic Analysis." *Lancet 375* (9727): 1704–20.

Shkolnikov, V., E. M. Andreev, D. A. Leon, M. McKee, F. Mesle, and J. Vallin. 2004. "Mortality Reversal in Russia: The Story So Far." *Hygiea Internationalis* 4: 29–80.

Shkolnikov, V., F. Mesle, and J. Vallin. 1996. "Health Crisis in Russia: Recent Trends in Life Expectancy and Causes of Death from 1970 to 1993." *Population: An English Selection* 8: 123–54.

Stillman, Steven. 2006. "Health and Nutrition in Eastern Europe and the Former Soviet Union during the Decade of Transition: A Review of the Literature." *Economics and Human Biology* 4 (1): 104–46.

Wang, H., L. Dwyer-Lindgren, K. T. Lofgren, J. K. Rajaratnam, J. R. Marcus, A. Levin-Rector, C. E. Levitz, A. D. Lopez, and C. J. L. Murray. 2012. "Age-Specific and Sex-Specific Mortality in 187 Countries, 1970–2010: A Systematic Analysis for the Global Burden of Disease Study 2010." *Lancet* 380 (9859): 2071–94.

World Bank. 2007. *Healthy Development: The World Bank Strategy for Health, Nutrition, and Population Results.* Washington, DC: World Bank.

———. 2012. *Golden Growth: Restoring the Luster of the European Economic Model.* Washington, DC: World Bank.

World Development Indicators (database). World Bank, Washington, DC. http://data.worldbank.org/data-catalog/world-development-indicators.

WHO (World Health Organization). National Health Accounts Database. 2012. World Health Organization, Geneva, http://www.who.int/nha/expenditure_database/en.

CHAPTER 2

Improving Welfare: The Value of Health

Key Messages

- The importance of improving health has been justified on the grounds that it is a basic human right, a central facet of human development, or a key determinant of happiness.

- The economic approach to the value of health and life is based on willingness to pay, and global estimates indicate that this is very high—in fact, high enough that over long periods of time, the value of health improvements has been similar in magnitude to the value of economic growth.

- The high value of life implies potentially high rates of return to health spending, even in the presence of large inefficiencies.

- There is some microeconomic evidence suggesting that better health has a positive impact on income, with the strongest evidence associated with early childhood health and nutrition. But there is only modest evidence of an impact of adult health on income, and in general, health impacts on income are not large enough to have a marked effect on economic growth.

- As such, the direct impact of health on welfare is a far more important channel than the productivity and growth impact for motivating policies aimed at improving health outcomes.

- Opinion survey evidence indicates that health sectors in ECA are consistently ranked as the top priority for additional government spending in most countries. Expectations for the government role in the health sector also appear very high.

- Health policy issues are likely to remain a population priority and prominent policy challenge for the foreseeable future as ECA aims for high-income status and beyond.

Why do we care about health? The answer may seem too obvious to be worthy of discussion. We all have an innate sense of why health matters. But at least some attempt to understand the value of better health is essential if we are to make progress on many important policy issues in the health sphere. While data on the costs of medical care are ubiquitous, there is comparatively less discussion of the benefits. Yet passing judgment on any policy or program requires some effort to address both. And while few people would disagree with the statement that people attach a high value to living long, healthy lives, the policy implications—both for how far this assertion can take us but also for its limits—are often not well understood.

Following the road map presented in chapter 1, we begin by looking at the relationship between health and overall welfare. As we will see, there is ample evidence—from economic theory, opinion polls, and elsewhere—that health matters enormously to well-being and is a major population priority. Taking some time to elaborate on this theme is important for putting into context the lack of health sector convergence between Europe and Central Asia (ECA) and Western Europe described in chapter 1 and to set the stage for the more in-depth exploration of the challenge of convergence in the chapters that follow.

Health Is a Major Determinant of Welfare

The relationship between health and welfare can be explored both directly, because health is closely connected to well-being, and indirectly, because better health may lead to a higher income and thus to the consumption of other goods that also matter for welfare. In this section, we begin with a focus on the direct impact, as it is the more important channel for motivating policies aimed at improving health outcomes. The health-income nexus, or investment value of health, is discussed briefly later in the section.

Health and Human Rights, Human Development, and Happiness

A common approach for asserting the importance of health is to state that it is a basic human "right." This view is affirmed in Article 25 of the Universal Declaration of Human Rights (1948). It is also expressed, in various ways, in the constitution of the World Health Organization (1946), the Alma-Ata Declaration on primary health care (1978), and Article 11 of the European Social Charter (1961). A commitment to health as a right—and sometimes explicitly as free access to medical care—is also enshrined in many national constitutions in the ECA region (Gotsadze and Gaal 2010). These documents put on paper what most people take as self-evident: that there is little more fundamental to our existence than our personal health.

Good health has also been closely associated with the very concept of "development." A prominent conceptual approach to human development has emphasized capabilities—in the simplest terms, focusing on what a person is able to do—and argued that development fundamentally entails overcoming capability deprivation (Sen 1985, 1999). In this sense, development is seen as a much broader process than just escaping from income poverty. As a means of expanding a person's capabilities, better physical and mental health plays an important role in this narrative. This notion contributed to the creation of the original United Nations (UN) Human Development Index, in which life expectancy featured as one of the four indicators.

Another rationale for affirming the importance of health can be drawn from the literature on "happiness." This research usually involves opinion surveys to identify the factors that contribute to a person's self-reported well-being. While there are debates about measurement, causality, and policy implications, here we simply note that these studies unsurprisingly show a strong relationship between health and happiness. In fact, it is often more statistically robust than the link between happiness and income (Graham 2008). Specifically in the context of ECA, the deterioration of public services such as health care has been identified as an important determinant of (un)happiness in transition countries (Guriev and Zhuravskaya 2009). In global studies of well-being, ECA countries stand out for their very low satisfaction with health, which in turn is associated with significantly lower life satisfaction (Deaton 2008).

Justifying health as a policy objective on the grounds that it is a basic human right, central to development, and a key determinant of happiness is an important argument that will resonate with many different audiences. But in the remainder of this section, we will shift our focus to the standard economic approach. It entails some possibly discomforting talk about the monetary value of health, but that approach is arguably well suited to a typical policy environment in which there are competing demands on limited resources. In many cases, this approach will lead to the same conclusion as the others—that health matters greatly—but it will also help identify some limits.

The Economic Approach: Pricing the Priceless

How much is a long, healthy life worth? The question itself may cause offense. Of course, there is no price tag on life, and if our health is in serious danger, we are often willing to pay "everything" to get better. The mere suggestion of attaching a monetary value to health outcomes can be controversial, but the reality is that such valuations do happen—often on a daily basis—when individuals and societies make decisions that involve a trade-off between health objectives and other benefits. Driving a car, eating certain types of food, or visiting a doctor all involve some kind of trade-off between potential health implications and other priorities, even if only implicitly.

One possible way to quantify the value of better health is to calculate the present value of all future earnings that are enabled by a particular state of health. In the extreme, the value of life itself would be summarized by the total economic output that a person produces during his or her lifetime. This approach, the "human capital method," emphasizes a person's productive potential. But it has the obvious drawback of attaching no value to the health of the elderly or others outside the labor force and sits uncomfortably with most people's perception of the value of life. In fact, it is not consistent with textbook welfare economics either, which is concerned with allocating resources (through compensation if necessary) to obtain the maximum well-being of individuals in society based on their own preferences (Drummond et al. 2005). Later in this chapter, we will return to the link between health and productivity, which is a legitimate policy question for understanding household income and economic growth. But it is not the appropriate yardstick for valuing better health. Nor, by extension, is it the correct way to assess the returns to public or private health spending (World Bank 1996).

How then do we assess the value of health? People want many things and have scarce resources with which to acquire them, and therefore some prioritization is necessary: we want to be healthy, but we do not want to spend everything we have on health. The value of health, then, can be interpreted as the amount of money we are willing to give up to achieve it, that is, our "willingness to pay." The challenge is the measurement problem: because better health is not available for sale at the market, estimating its value is not easy. Box 2.1 elaborates.

The basic finding that emerges from research on this topic is, not surprisingly, that the value of life is very high. In probability terms, people are willing to pay amounts well in excess of their annual income, in fact, at least five times as much, for additional years of life. Moreover, these estimates tend to be conservative, since they focus on the gains from reduced mortality risk but not reduced morbidity.

At this point, it is worth pausing for a reality check. Does the finding that people are willing to pay dearly (in forgone consumption) for improved odds of a long life in good health ring true? In other words, do these very high estimates of the value of life make sense? It is helpful to reflect on how these results align with our basic intuition.

One way to check the plausibility of research-based estimates of the value of life is to ask people to choose hypothetically between the health and income levels that prevailed during different historical periods (Nordhaus 2003). A variant of this approach was tested with over 6,000 survey respondents across six countries in ECA (Azerbaijan, Georgia, Moldova, the Russian Federation, Tajikistan, and Uzbekistan). People were asked to choose whether they would prefer to live in a country with an average income of US$500 per month and a life expectancy of 80 years, or in another country with an average income of US$2,500 per month and a life expectancy of 70 years. Roughly speaking, this corresponds to choosing between a leap forward from the health and wealth of ECA today to *either* the average income of the EU-15 *or* its average life span, but not both. The question was asked in both numeric and general terms. The results indicate that people are almost equally divided between wanting to be five times richer and having a life span that is 10 years longer (figure 2.1). This finding lends further support to assumptions about a high value on life.

BOX 2.1

What Is Better Health Worth? Introducing the Value of Statistical Life

There are two basic approaches to estimating a person's willingness to pay for better health. The first is the stated-preference (or contingent valuation) method, which involves asking a person to choose between various options as a typical consumer would. For example, a respondent could be asked whether he or she would be willing to pay US$10,000 for a heart operation that, on average, results in two additional years of life. The problem is that the respondent is facing a hypothetical situation—no real transaction takes place. The alternative is the revealed preference approach, which focuses on actual individual behaviors in economic decision making. For example, one can look at market outcomes such as the wage premium necessary to attract workers to take a job with some risk of personal injury or the amount that consumers are willing to pay for safety devices such as automobile air bags or smoke detectors (Drummond et al. 2005).

The result of these analyses is a concept called the value of statistical life (VSL). It is defined as the amount required to accept additional risk (or pay for lower risk) divided by the level of that risk. In essence, it tells us how much people would be willing to pay for small increases in the odds of survival. Thus, a key aspect of willingness-to-pay analysis is that it takes a probabilistic approach to the value of health. Asking people how much they would pay to avoid a fate of certain death would not yield useful insights—nor is it realistic. Our everyday decisions about food, transport, work, or medical care are made in a context of uncertainty. Therefore, valuing health can be seen as equivalent to asking how much people are willing to pay for better odds of surviving in good health.

For society as a whole, a policy expected to "save" a statistical life is one that is predicted to result in one less death within the population over a certain time period. In this case, as for many policies, the individuals whose lives would be extended cannot be identified in advance. As such, it is not the same as saving a specific person from certain death. The link with health spending should be clear: investing in the health system can be seen as a collective effort to reduce population-wide mortality rates through access to better medical care. The extent to which a society is willing to pay taxes to fund its health system will thus in part reflect VSL.

A large number of studies have been undertaken to estimate VSL among people of different ages, at different income levels, and across different countries. A widely cited literature review estimated a VSL between US$3 million and US$7 million in the United States, for an average of around US$5 million (Viscusi 1993). This amount can be translated into a value of a statistical life *year*, for example, of US$250,000 for a middle-aged adult in the United States. Cross-country studies have helped identify a range for the income elasticity of VSL or, more simplistically, a typical value of about 120 times gross domestic product (GDP) per capita (Miller 2000; Viscusi and Aldy 2003). In ECA, this number translates into between US$250,000 and over US$3 million (purchasing power parity), depending on the country. The value of additional life-years would

continued

BOX 2.1 *continued*

accordingly range approximately from US$10,000 to US$170,000, or at least five times income per capita. While VSL is implied to be lower among poorer populations, the average value within a country can be seen as a guide to society's willingness to pay for an equitable health financing system that enables access to care for all.

The imprecise nature of VSL estimates may appear to render this concept unhelpful for policy purposes. But, in fact, the results are accurate enough that many health interventions can be either "ruled in" or "ruled out"—that is, worth the cost or not—on the basis of VSL estimates. In fact, VSL is applied by government agencies in some countries, such as the United States. We explore this idea further below.

FIGURE 2.1

The Value of Extra Years of Life Relative to Extra Income Is High

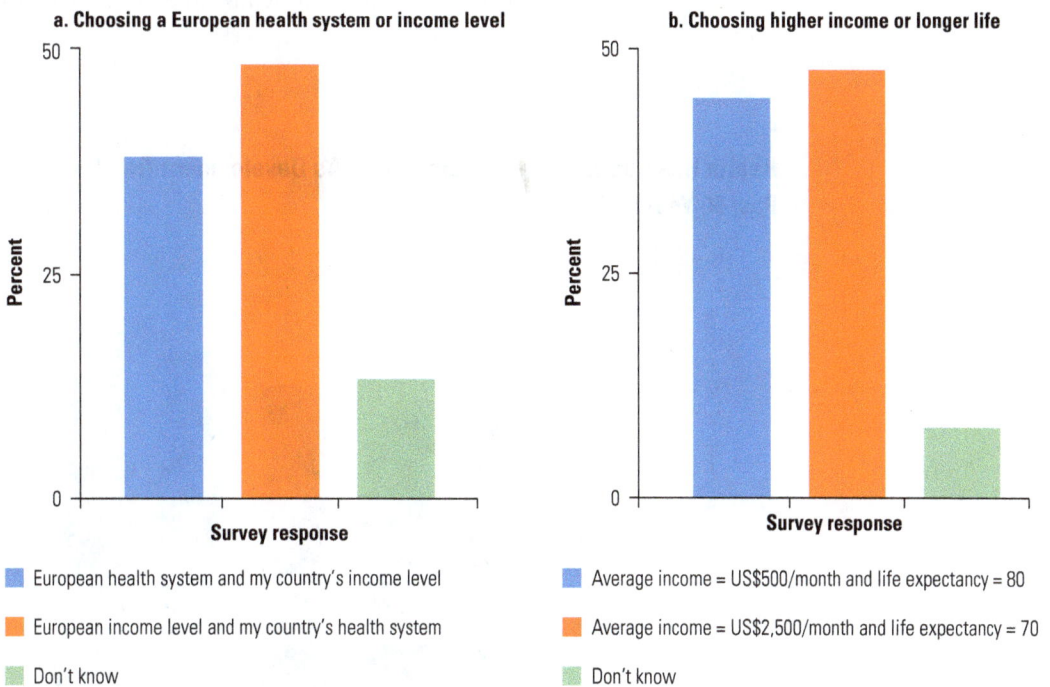

a. Choosing a European health system or income level

b. Choosing higher income or longer life

- European health system and my country's income level
- European income level and my country's health system
- Don't know

- Average income = US$500/month and life expectancy = 80
- Average income = US$2,500/month and life expectancy = 70
- Don't know

Source: World Bank 2012.
Note: The survey question asked of residents of Europe and Central Asia was "In which country would you rather live?" with a choice of responses as shown.

What Does a High Value of Life and Health Imply for ECA?

Three major implications for ECA's health policies emerge from the foregoing discussion of the value of life and from the broader research literature it has spawned during the past decade. First, it reinforces the key message from chapter 1 that ECA's long-term health outcome performance has been weak by global standards. To illustrate, we use the concept of "full income," which combines gross domestic product (GDP) per capita and life expectancy—or, put differently, the quality and quantity of life—into a single measure of overall welfare. Full income growth is measured by adding the value of changes in annual mortality (based on value of statistical life [VSL]) to changes in annual GDP per capita. Figure 2.2 applies the methodology developed in a well-known study to compare the contribution of health to the growth of full income in ECA with the corresponding figures for the other five World Bank regions between 1960 and 2008 (Becker, Philipson, and Soares 2005). It shows that less than 10 percent of ECA's full income growth since 1960 can be attributed to health improvements, by far the lowest share in the six regions (albeit from a higher baseline). Even more broadly, ECA's development underperformance due to slow health gains also stands out when leisure and inequality are added to consumption and health in a single welfare metric (Jones and Klenow 2011).

FIGURE 2.2

Health Has Contributed Very Little to ECA's Development Trend in the Past 50 Years

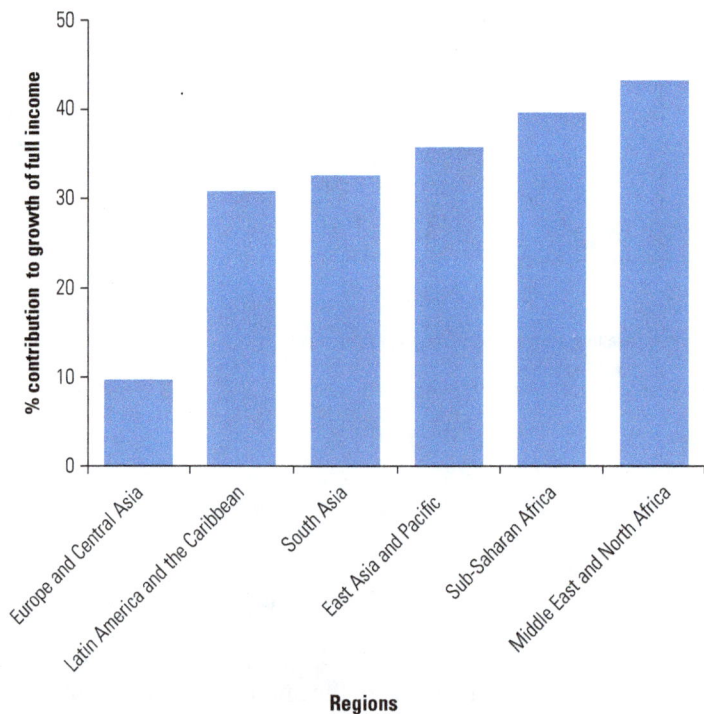

Source: Calculations based on Becker, Philipson, and Soares 2005.
Note: Figure shows the contribution of health to the growth of "full income," 1960–2008. ECA = Europe and Central Asia.

Reconsidering the Returns to Health Spending

A second implication is that the historical growth of health spending in advanced countries has on average been "worth it." A lot of money has been spent on health, but people are living longer, healthier lives in no small part due to the improvements in medical care that this spending has helped bring about. For a Western European, an equivalent question to the one asked in figure 2.1 is whether he or she would prefer an additional US$3,000 per year (total per capita health spending has increased from roughly US$500 to US$3,500 between 1960 and 2010), while accepting a 1960s health system, or if he or she would prefer to forgo the money in return for today's health system and outcomes. Many would find this choice difficult.

More precisely, rates of return to health spending on specific conditions have far exceeded what is typically expected of private or public investment in other spheres. Table 2.1 shows some examples of rates of return to spending on specific conditions in the United States. This has important implications for the discussion of efficiency in chapter 5. On aggregate, it has been estimated that the gains from improved health outcomes have equaled or exceeded the total value of all measured economic growth in the United States both over the course of the 20th century (Nordhaus 2003) and since 1970 (Murphy and Topel 2006).

It is important to note that the high average value on health spending in rich countries does not contradict the commonly held view that these systems are also inefficient. The key distinction is whether we are talking about *some* or *all* health care as being wasteful. This point is explored further in chapter 5. While table 2.1 shows the most favorable returns, there are certain procedures that do not appear to offer good value for money (for example, treatment of

TABLE 2.1

High Rates of Return on Many Health Care Services in the United States

Condition or Treatment	Benefit-to-Cost Ratio Based on VSL
Anti-hypertensive therapy	10 to 1 for men; 6 to 1 for women
Heart attack treatments	7 to 1
Medical management of coronary heart disease	6 to 1
Low birthweight infant care	6 to 1
Breast and colon cancer screening	> 1
Lung cancer treatment	< 1

Sources: Cutler and McClellan 2001; Cutler et al. 2007; Rosen et al. 2007; Cutler 2008.
Note: VSL = value of statistical life.

lung cancer). The concept of VSL—unlike, for example, a rights-based approach to health—can help us identify what portion of health spending is "worth it" as well as those components that are not.

The third implication of the value-of-life estimates is that in the future, ECA also has the potential to achieve high rates of return on health spending, just as advanced countries have done during recent decades. ECA's life expectancy today is similar to the EU-15's during the 1960s, and thus if countries were to repeat the health spending growth *and* the life expectancy gains that have been achieved in the West over the past 50 years, they should achieve good value for money. But caution is warranted here, since such an outcome would of course depend on well-functioning health systems, an issue that will be discussed at length later in this report. Otherwise, increased health spending could be wasted. In fact, ECA should aim to achieve the same outcomes at less cost than the EU-15 through more efficient health systems. Last, the potentially high rates of return to health spending discussed here do not address the issue of whether such expenditures should be public or private. That will be addressed further in chapters 4 and 5.

As we look further into the future, it is also worth noting that as countries grow richer, the value of health improvements becomes ever larger. In economic jargon, while the marginal utility of consumption declines, the marginal utility of longer life does not. People would prefer extra years of life in which to enjoy current living standards to more consumption compressed into a fixed life span. When a country is rich enough that additional consumption is likely to be for an extra car or vacation, the relative value of, say, a hip replacement or surgery that can be expected to extend life by a year will be far higher than if basic needs or consumer durables are beyond reach for a large share of households. While this eventuality may be a long way off for many ECA countries, the evolution of preferences does help explain why health spending tends to rise relentlessly as a share of GDP. The implication is that an increasing proportion of a (growing) economy allocated to health is fully consistent with welfare maximization. It has even been suggested that health spending would optimally rise to 30 percent of GDP in a country as rich as the United States in the year 2050 (Hall and Jones 2007).

In sum, the direct contribution of health improvements to overall welfare is very large. In many countries (but not ECA as a whole), the value of decades of health improvements has been of a similar magnitude to decades of consumption gains enabled by economic growth. As a result, the total benefit of health care spending has sometimes far exceeded its costs in advanced countries, even in the presence of significant waste. As noted at the outset, it is important to acknowledge the value of health if we are going to make progress with the fundamental policy issues confronting the sector.

Health Can Affect Productivity and Growth, but There Is Only a Modest Link

How much does better health matter for economic performance? Intuitively, we know that being in a state of poor health will have an impact on our productive potential, whether we are working in an office or in a field. But the size of the impact, and how much it matters in aggregate, is less clear. With a shrinking labor force due to aging, many ECA countries are looking for ways to encourage work at older ages. Self-assessed health among the 50- to 65-year-old cohort is lower in ECA than in Western Europe. With this factor in mind, we shift our attention to the indirect link between health improvements and overall welfare through its effect on income and growth. That link may be referred to as the "investment value of health," as opposed to the consumption value, as discussed earlier.

In theory, improved health can affect income through various mechanisms. Better health in childhood has been shown to improve physiological and cognitive development, which can lead to better educational outcomes, greater human capital accumulation, and higher productivity and income later in life (Grossman 1972). Health can affect income of adults in several ways. First, labor productivity may improve if healthier individuals are more physically and mentally productive or more effective at using technology or resources (Currie and Madrian 1999). Second, healthy adults may be less likely to miss work due to illness, thereby increasing their earnings. Finally, healthier adults may invest more in their own and their children's human capital because they expect to enjoy longer, healthier lives. Greater human capital accumulation through higher investments can then result in higher income (Grossman 2000).

Unfortunately, several factors complicate research on the relationship between health and income, including measurement issues, reverse causality, and unobservable factors. Neither mortality-based indicators nor subjective self-assessments of health status may adequately capture the link between health and productivity (Schultz 2005). The two-way relationship between health and income also complicates empirical research, because studies that find correlations between health and income often cannot determine whether higher-income individuals invest more in their health or whether healthier individuals are able to earn higher incomes. Furthermore, there may be unobservable factors such as living conditions or education that affect both health and income. Thus, better health may be correlated with higher income not by a direct causal relationship but by a third factor that is driving both.

As a result, there has been significant debate about the existence of a causal relationship between health and income. Studies vary widely with respect to methodology and data quality, with a mix of "rigorous scientific investigation and well-motivated advocacy" (Jack and Lewis 2009). Researchers have used microeconomic data, simulations, economic theory, cross-country analysis, and experimental evidence. Literature reviews on the relationship have arrived at similar conclusions (Kremer and Glennerster 2012; Bleakley 2010a; Spence and Lewis 2009; Currie 2009; Strauss and Thomas 2007). First, there is some microeconomic evidence suggesting an impact of health on income, with the strongest evidence from early childhood health and nutrition. Second, these microeconomic estimates are not large enough to indicate that improving health will lead to large macroeconomic impacts. Third, cross-country macroeconomic studies do not provide convincing evidence of an impact. A brief summary of the literature is presented in box 2.2, drawn from background work undertaken for this report (Yeh 2012).

Last, it should also be noted that while there is little robust evidence that health causes growth, it does not appear that income per se has a significant causal impact on health outcomes (Cutler, Deaton, and Lleras-Muney 2006). While *levels* of income and health outcomes are strongly correlated, as shown in chapter 1, there is almost no relationship between rates of economic growth and changes in life expectancy during the past 50 years (Deaton 2007). Instead, it would appear that some third factor—such as education at the individual level and institutional capacity at the country level—is likely to play a significant determining role in both health improvement and income growth.

In sum, while there is some evidence that ill health can have a negative impact on productivity and income, especially in the context of early childhood, the overall impact is not major. The main effect of health on welfare is the direct impact described earlier, not the indirect channel (through income) discussed here.

Health Is a Public Priority Here to Stay

The previous section established the high value of health as seen through various conceptual frameworks. But there is abundant evidence from less abstract sources that health concerns figure

BOX 2.2

Searching for the Impact of Health on Income

The strongest available microeconomic evidence on the impact of health on income relates to *early childhood health and nutrition.* While mortality in ECA is largely due to other causes, childhood health and nutrition remain a key issue, particularly in Central Asia and among the Roma population of Central and Eastern Europe. The public health literature has explored the impact of maternal and child undernutrition on a variety of outcomes, including stunting, cognitive development, education, productivity, and income (Grantham-McGregor et al. 2007; Victora et al. 2008). It has found positive associations but not causal impacts, between birthweight, child size, and income. Experimental and quasi-experimental studies have also established a clear relationship among child health, educational attainment, and adult earnings (Miguel and Kremer 2004; Almond 2006).

In general, the microeconomic literature on the impact of *adult health* on income remains suggestive, especially for noncommunicable diseases. Many studies find positive correlations between adult health and labor supply or earnings but often do not adequately control for confounding factors (Bleakley 2010a; Strauss and Thomas 2007). Robust evaluations of adult health interventions and income are rare. Some suggestive evidence of an impact of adult health on labor supply and productivity can be found in ECA. In Russia, adult health status is positively associated with labor force participation, but not with wages or hours worked (Schultz 2008). Elsewhere, studies of 14 ECA countries and Western Europe found that better self-reported health measures were correlated with increased labor supply and productivity, but not always (Suhrcke et al. 2008; Suhrcke, Rocco, and McKee 2007).

Much of the literature on adult health and income focuses on specific behavioral risk factors such as excessive *alcohol consumption, smoking, or obesity.* The effect of alcohol on income is ambiguous. A positive relationship between alcohol consumption and labor participation was found in Russia, with a negative effect only for binge drinking (Schultz 2008). Overall, a review of the literature suggests that alcohol use does not have a substantial negative effect on either labor supply or productivity except in the case of alcoholism or problem drinking (Lye and Hirschberg 2010). Smoking can negatively affect income in several ways, most significantly as smokers may have increased health problems, leading to greater absenteeism or lower productivity while on the job. The empirical evidence suggests that smoking is strongly correlated with reduced wages. Studies in Albania, Canada, and the United States find lower wages among smokers than nonsmokers, but these do not establish causality (Lokshin and Beegle 2006; Levine, Gustafson, and Valenchik 1997; Auld 2005). Studies on obesity find a small negative relationship between body mass index and income for females and no relationship or a slightly positive one for males (Cawley 2004; Gregory and Ruhm 2011; Lindeboom, Lundborg, and van der Klaauw 2010). For example, Huffman and Rizov (2011) examine Russian data from 1994 to

continued

BOX 2.2 *continued*

2005 and show no evidence of lower wages due to a higher body mass index but do find slightly reduced labor supply among the very overweight and obese.

While the microeconomic literature finds some substantial impacts of health on income at the individual level, recent studies have shown that these findings do not translate into large macroeconomic impacts. Microeconomic studies typically do not account for general equilibrium effects, which are important because health investments that increase individual worker productivity cannot be assumed to do so at the same rate for the entire population. Fixed resources, increasing population growth due to better health, diminishing returns to labor, or other factors can change the estimated effect of health on income when aggregated to a macro-level (Acemoglu and Johnson 2007).

If these general equilibrium effects are not accounted for, the estimates of the impact on GDP can appear quite large. For example, Suhrcke et al. (2007) calculate that gradually reducing mortality rates from noncommunicable diseases in Russia down to those in the EU-15 from 2002 to 2025 would lead to an increase in GDP of 3.6–4.8 percent. Lokshin and Beegle (2006) also estimated a large impact of smoking on GDP. But when general equilibrium effects are taken into account, the effects on GDP are greatly reduced (Weil 2007; Ashraf, Lester, and Weil 2009; Bleakley 2010b).

The weakest evidence on health and income is from cross-country macroeconomic studies, because of their inability to control for endogeneity and unobserved characteristics. Richer countries typically have healthier populations, and it is difficult at a country level to distinguish why. Many other factors such as institutional quality, education, governance, and poverty affect both health and income and often through the reverse channel of income to health. Recent literature reviews have found the cross-country literature to be unconvincing, owing to methodological issues (Kremer and Glennerster 2012; Bleakley 2010a; Spence and Lewis 2009).

prominently in the lives of populations across ECA. This section looks at a range of opinion poll evidence from across the continent and considers what it means for the health sector going forward. It concludes by stepping back and briefly considering the politics of health spending.

We begin with population views on government spending priorities. Across the region, over 50,000 survey respondents in two rounds (2006 and 2010) of the Life in Transition Survey (EBRD 2010) were asked the following question: In your opinion, which of these fields should be the first and second priorities for extra government spending? The results were remarkably consistent. Health is identified as the top priority for additional government investment in over 75 percent (22 of 29) of the countries in ECA (figure 2.3). This

FIGURE 2.3

Health Is a Top Priority for Populations across the Region, 2010

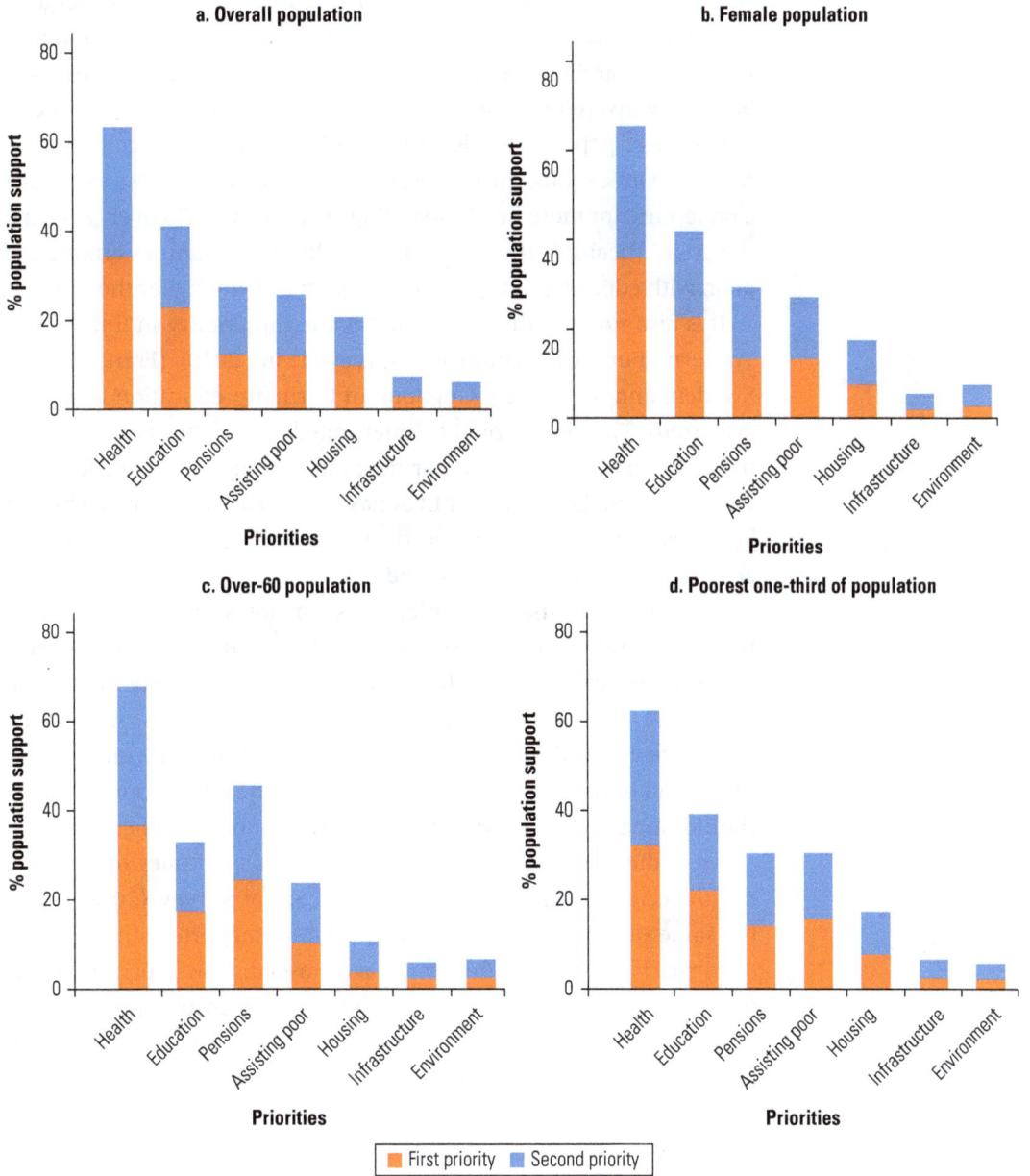

Source: EBRD 2010.
Note: Figure shows the top priorities for government investment in Europe and Central Asia.

outcome was the same in both 2010 and 2006, despite the intervening economic crisis, so it appears to be an enduring sentiment.
The countries in which another priority was placed higher than
health in 2010 were Albania, Azerbaijan, Croatia, Kosovo, Serbia,
Tajikistan, and Turkey.

This preference is also a few percentage points stronger among women than men (although it is still the top priority among men, too). Among the elderly population (over 60), additional health spending was preferred to more pension spending in 26 of 29 countries and by a significant margin across the region as a whole. This generation may be acutely aware of the loss of the (free) pretransition health system, but younger populations also prioritize health. Finally, segmenting by socioeconomic status, the poorest third of the population also expressed a preference for more health spending by a wide margin over "assisting the poor" (health is the top priority in 20 of 29 countries among the poor, with education and assisting the poor accounting for the rest).

It is also noteworthy that health is the top priority in four of five Western European countries surveyed in 2010 (France, Italy, Sweden, and the United Kingdom; in Germany, education is slightly preferred). This result could be interpreted as evidence that no country can hope to satisfy popular demands for more health spending. But it may also be a sign that ECA has reached a stage at which health becomes a permanent fixture on the policy agenda and to which governments will need to respond.

Of course, population preferences do not amount to the only word on optimal budget allocations—far from it. In many cases, performance can and should be improved by making better use of existing resources, as will be discussed in later chapters. And policy makers have the difficult task of taking into account a wide array of issues and balancing many competing demands. But popular views should nonetheless be an important voice in those deliberations.

An additional piece of evidence on popular attitudes toward the health sector comes from the European Social Survey (2008) (with the same questions asked by a World Bank–supported survey in six countries farther east). Individuals were asked, How much responsibility do you think governments should have to ensure: (a) adequate health care for the sick? (b) a reasonable standard of living for the old? (c) a job for everyone who wants one? Answers were given on a scale of 0–10 (figure 2.4).

The results indicate that an overwhelming share of respondents in the Commonwealth of Independent States (CIS) region view all three issues—especially health care and old age security, but also jobs—to be predominantly the responsibility of government. When contrasted with other regions, it would appear that expectations of government are *too* high and that, over time, people will need to recognize their own responsibilities. In health care, this will include, among other things, addressing risky behaviors and the need for self-management of chronic disease.

FIGURE 2.4

High Expectations of Government in the Health Sector

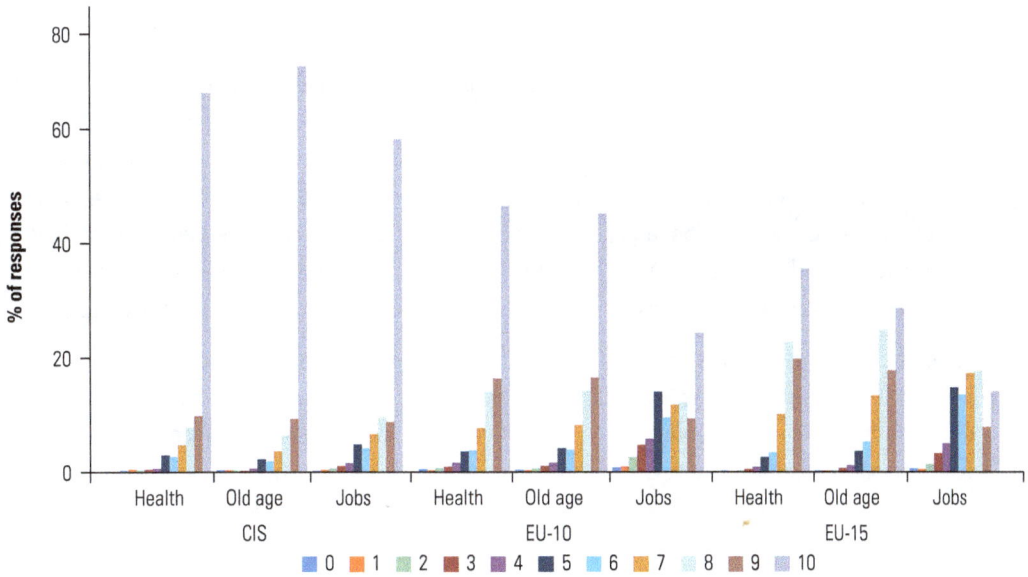

Sources: European Social Survey 2008; World Bank 2012.
Note: Figure shows how survey respondents perceive the responsibility of government on a scale of 0 (no government role expected) to 10 (a very strong role is expected). Responses are shown independently for each region of residence and sector (health, old age, and jobs). CIS = Commonwealth of Independent States.

But the profile of responses in the EU-15 also points to the enduring *relative* importance attached to government responsibility in the health sector. In these countries, it is judged to be higher than for old-age security or jobs. This ranking may reflect the person-on-the-street's interpretation of what policy makers know as extensive market failures and the complexity of choices in the sector. People don't want to be left alone to navigate medical care and insurance markets in search of a product for which both need and quality are difficult to ascertain, that could be life saving or bank breaking (or both or neither), and that obliges them to engage with people who may or may not have their best interests at heart.

In sum, survey evidence suggests that the health sector is a key concern of populations across ECA. It is consistently viewed as the top priority for government investment, and a very high degree of responsibility for the sector is assigned to governments. As such, it is likely that the challenges to be addressed in the remainder of this report will stay on the policy agenda, in one form or another, for many years to come. This also means that health will figure more prominently in elections (box 2.3). As middle-income countries strive to reach high-income status, the health sector's role in the development agenda would seem destined only to grow in importance.

BOX 2.3

The Changing Politics of Health Spending

One question that arises from the discussion so far is why health budgets do not increase if the popular view is that health is the top priority for additional spending and, moreover, largely the responsibility of government. While this report will focus primarily on the economic and public health aspects of the sector, it is worth taking a moment to consider the politics. There is no clear-cut answer to this question, and so here we will provide only a brief overview of the existing literature. A key finding is that public spending priorities may be biased against health under the circumstances currently prevailing in many ECA countries, for a number of possible reasons.

One strand of the literature has emphasized factors related to democracy and accountability. For example, cross-country research has found that public investment spending (for example, on infrastructure) is higher in countries with weak governance and minimal political competition, possibly because capital projects become vehicles for rent seeking where governance is weak (Keefer and Knack 2007). This leaves less budget room for health and other social sectors. Another argument put forward is that political pressures to raise spending on broad-based services such as health and education are weak in political environments characterized by social fragmentation or a lack of information about politicians' performance and their credibility. Under these circumstances, other sectors are preferred by self-serving politicians (Keefer and Khemani 2005). Yet another line of reasoning is that governments prefer to spend on "visible" expenditure types—those that are more easily observed and measured, as well as less complex—in nascent democracies. It is argued that health is among the least-visible sectors, due to the complexity of its production function (Mani and Mukand 2007). Instead, cash benefits, pensions, or capital projects may be preferred. Other work has also highlighted how democracy can provide a boost to the health sector (Besley and Kudamatsu 2006).

There is some empirical evidence from ECA to support these arguments. Since 1997, the budget share allocated to health has declined steeply in countries deemed "not free" by Freedom House, declined slightly in "partly free" countries, and increased in "free" ECA countries. There is also a positive correlation between these budget trends and measures of good governance (Kaufman and Kraay 2011). But, as always, correlation does not imply causation.

Another strand of the literature has emphasized the role of women's voice. Evidence from settings as diverse as the United States in the early 20th century and India today suggests that the role of women in politics can affect budget allocations related to health investments (Miller 2008; Chattopadhyay and Duflo 2004). Two of ECA's lowest health spenders, Armenia and Georgia, also have among the lowest proportions of female parliamentarians in the region (Inter-Parliamentary Union 2012).

Of course, more spending on other sectors results in less for health, and military spending offers an example. Many of the countries that experienced conflict in the 1990s—such as

continued

Armenia, Azerbaijan, Georgia, and Tajikistan—all continue to allocate relatively smaller budget shares to health, in part because expenditures on defense, public order, and safety are significantly higher than in other countries in the region.

But as countries become more developed both politically and economically, and these other factors subside, the role of the health sector in politics is likely to become increasingly prominent. It is not difficult to find specific examples of elections in which health issues were a key campaign issue in higher-income countries. The unpopular introduction of copayments helped oust the sitting Slovak government in its 2006 election. In Hungary, a referendum on the introduction of copayments was held in 2008. Health reform was a top issue in the U.S. midterm congressional elections in 2010. Indeed, in high-income OECD countries between 1971 and 2004, health spending tended to increase more during election years, regardless of the political stripes of the incumbent party (that is, whether it was Left or Right) (Potrafke 2010). Presumably, politicians judged it to be a winner. Thus, whatever one thinks of the technocratic merits of health policies, the politics of health spending are likely to figure more prominently and tip the balance in favor of more spending over time.

References

Acemoglu, Daron, and Simon Johnson. 2007. "Disease and Development: The Effect of Life Expectancy on Economic Growth." *Journal of Political Economy* 115 (6): 925–85.

Almond, Douglas. 2006. "Is the 1918 Influenza Pandemic Over? Long-Term Effects of in Utero Influenza Exposure in the Post-1940 U.S. Population." *Journal of Political Economy* 114 (4): 672–712.

Ashraf, Quamrul H., Ashley Lester, and David N. Weil. 2009. "When Does Improving Health Raise GDP?" In *NBER Macroeconomics Annual 23*, edited by Daron Acemoglu, Kenneth Rogoff, and Michael Woodford, 157–204. Cambridge, MA: National Bureau of Economic Research.

Auld, M. Christopher. 2005. "Smoking, Drinking and Income." *Journal of Human Resources* 40 (2): 505–18.

Becker, G. S., T. J. Philipson, and R. R. Soares. 2005. "The Quantity and Quality of Life and the Evolution of World Inequality." *American Economic Review* 95 (1): 277–91.

Besley, T., and M. Kudamatsu. 2006. "Health and Democracy." *American Economic Review* 96 (2): 313–18.

Bleakley, Hoyt. 2010a. "Health, Human Capital, and Development." *Annual Review of Economics* 2: 283–310.

———. 2010b. "Malaria Eradication in the Americas: A retrospective Analysis of Childhood Exposure." *American Economic Journal: Applied* 2 (2): 1–45.

Cawley, John. 2004. "The Impact of Obesity on Wages." *Journal of Human Resources* 39 (2): 451–74.

Chattopadhyay, R., and E. Duflo. 2004. "Women as Policy Makers: Evidence from a Randomized Policy Experiment in India." *Econometrica* 75 (5): 1409–43.

Currie, Janet. 2009. "Healthy, Wealthy, and Wise: Socioeconomic Status, Poor Health in Childhood, and Human Capital Development." *Journal of Economic Literature* 47 (1): 87–122.

Currie, Janet, and Bridgette C. Madrian. 1999. "Health, Health Insurance and the Labour Market." In *Handbook of Labour Economics,* edited by Orley Ashenfelter and David Card, 2209–3415. Amsterdam: Elsevier Science BV.

Cutler, D. M. 2008. "Are We Finally Winning the War on Cancer?" *Journal of Economic Perspectives* 22 (4): 3–26.

Cutler, D. M., A. Deaton, and A. Lleras-Muney. 2006. "The Determinants of Mortality." *Journal of Economic Perspectives* 20 (3): 97–120.

Cutler, D. M., and M. McClellan. 2001. "Is Technological Change in Medicine Worth It?" *Health Affairs* 20 (5): 11–29.

Cutler, D. M., G. Long, E. Berndt, J. Royer, A. Fournier, A. Sasser, and P. Cremieux. 2007. "The Value of Antihypertensive Drugs: A Perspective on Medical Innovation." *Health Affairs* 26 (1): 97–110.

Deaton, A. 2007. "Global Patterns of Income and Health: Facts, Interpretations, and Policies." UNU-WIDER Lecture, September 26, 2006, Princeton University, http://www.princeton.edu/rpds/papers/pdfs/deaton_WIDER_annual-lecture-2006.pdf.

———. 2008. "Income, Health, and Well-Being around the World: Evidence from the Gallup World Poll." *Journal of Economic Perspectives* 22 (2): 53–72.

Drummond, M. F., M. Sculpher, G. Torrance, B. O'Brien, and G. Stoddart. 2005. *Methods for the Economic Evaluation of Health Care Programs.* 3rd ed. Oxford: Oxford University Press.

EBRD (European Bank for Reconstruction and Development). 2010. *Life in Transition Survey,* http://www.ebrd.com/pages/research/publications/special/transitionII.shtml.

European Social Survey. 2008. Round 4 data file edition 4.1. Norwegian Social Science Data Services, Norway—Data Archive and distributor of ESS data.

Gotsadze, G., and P. Gaal. 2010. "Coverage Decisions: Benefit Entitlements and Patient Cost Sharing." In *Implementing Health Financing Reform: Lessons from Countries in Transition,* edited by Joseph Kutzin, Cheryl Cashin, and Melitta Jakab, 187–217. Copenhagen: World Health Organization.

Graham, C. 2008. "Happiness and Health: Lessons—and Questions—for Public Policy." *Health Affairs* 27 (1): 72–87.

Grantham-McGregor, Sally, Yin Bun Cheung, Santiago Cueto, Paul Glewwe, Linda Richter, Barbara Strupp, and the International Child Development Steering Group. 2007. "Developmental Potential in the First 5 Years for Children in Developing Countries." *Lancet* 369: 60–70.

Gregory, Christian A., and Christopher J. Ruhm. 2011. "Where Does the Wage Penalty Bite?" In *Economic Aspects of Obesity,* edited by Michael Grossman and Naci H. Mocan, 315–47. Cambridge, MA: National Bureau of Economic Research.

Grossman, Michael. 1972. "On the Concept of Health Capital and the Demand for Health." *Journal of Political Economy* 80 (2): 223–55.

———. 2000. "The Human Capital Model." In *Handbook of Health Economics*, vol. 1, edited by Anthony J. Culyer and Joseph P. Newhouse, 347–408. Amsterdam: Elsevier.

Guriev, S., and E. Zhuravskaya. 2009. "(Un)Happiness in Transition." *Journal of Economic Perspectives* 23 (2): 143–68.

Hall, R. E., and C. I. Jones. 2007. "The Value of Life and the Rise in Health Spending." *Quarterly Journal of Economics* 122 (1): 39–72.

Huffman, Sonya, and Marian Rizov. 2011. "Body Weight and Labour Market Outcomes in Post-Soviet Russia." Working Paper 11007, Iowa State University, Ames, Iowa.

Inter-Parliamentary Union. 2012. http://www.ipu.org/wmn-e/world-arc.htm.

Jack, William, and Maureen Lewis. 2009. "Health Investments and Economic Growth: Macroeconomic Evidence and Microeconomic Foundation." In *Health and Growth*, edited by Michael Spence and Maureen Lewis, 1–39. Washington, DC: Commission on Growth and Development, World Bank.

Jones, C. I., and P. Klenow. 2011. "Beyond GDP: Welfare across Countries and Time." NBER Working Paper 16352, National Bureau of Economic Research, Cambridge, MA.

Kaufmann, D., and A. Kraay. 2011. World Governance Indicators (database). World Bank, Washington, DC, http://info.worldbank.org/governance/wgi/index.asp.

Keefer, P., and S. Khemani. 2005. "Democracy, Public Expenditures, and the Poor." *World Bank Research Observer* 20: 1–27.

Keefer, P., and S. Knack. 2007. "Boondoggles, Rent-Seeking, and Political Checks and Balances: Public Investment under Unaccountable Governments." *Review of Economics and Statistics* 89 (3): 566–72.

Kremer, Michael, and Rachel Glennerster. 2012. "Improving Health in Developing Countries: Evidence from Randomized Evaluations." In *Handbook of Health Economics*, edited by Mark V. Pauly, Thomas G. McGuire, and Pedro P. Barros, 201–315. Oxford: Elsevier Science BV.

Levine, Phillip B., Tara A. Gustafson, and Ann D. Valenchik. 1997. "More Bad News for Smokers? The Effects of Cigarette Smoking on Wages." *Industrial and Labor Relations Review* 50: 493–509.

Lindeboom, Maarten, Petter Lundborg, and Bas van der Klaauw. 2010. "Assessing the Impact of Obesity on Labor Market Outcomes." *Economics & Human Biology* 8 (3): 309–19.

Lokshin, Michael, and Kathleen Beegle. 2006. "Forgone Earnings from Smoking: Evidence for a Developing Country." Policy Research Working Paper 4018, World Bank, Washington, DC.

Lye, Jenny, and Joe Hirschberg. 2010. "Alcohol Consumption and Human Capital: A Retrospective Study of the Literature." *Journal of Economic Surveys* 24 (2): 309–38.

Mani, A., and S. Mukand. 2007. "Democracy, Visibility, and Public Good Provision." *Journal of Development Economics* 83: 506–29.

Miguel, Edward, and Michael Kremer. 2004. "Worms: Identifying Impacts on Education and Health in the Presence of Treatment Externalities." *Econometrica* 72 (1): 159–217.

Miller, Grant. 2008. "Women's Suffrage, Political Responsiveness, and Child Survival in American History." *Quarterly Journal of Economics* 123 (3): 1287–1327.

Miller, T. R. 2000. "Variations between Countries in Values of Statistical Life." *Journal of Transport Economics and Policy* 34 (2): 169–88.

Murphy K .M., and R. H. Topel. 2006. "The Value of Health and Longevity." *Journal of Political Economy* 114 (5): 871–904.

Nordhaus, W. D. 2003. "The Health of Nations: The Contribution of Improved Health to Living Standards." In *Measuring the Gains from Medical Research: An Economic Approach*, edited by K. M. Murphy and R. H. Topel, 9–40. Chicago: University of Chicago Press.

Potrafke, N. 2010. "The Growth of Public Health Expenditures in OECD Countries: Do Government Ideology and Electoral Motives Matter?" *Journal of Health Economics* 29 (6): 797–810.

Rosen, A., D. Cutler, D. Rosen, H. Hu, and S. Vijan. 2007. "The Value of Coronary Heart Disease Care for the Elderly: 1987–2002." *Health Affairs* 26 (1): 111–23.

Schultz, T. Paul. 2005. "Productive Benefits of Health: Evidence from Low-Income Countries." Yale Economic Growth Center Discussion Paper 903, Yale University, New Haven, CT.

———. 2008. "Health Disabilities and Labor Productivity in Russia in 2004: Health Consequences beyond Premature Death." In *Economic Implications of Chronic Illness and Disability in Eastern Europe and the Former Soviet Union*, edited by Cem Mete, 85–118. Washington, DC: World Bank.

Sen, Amartya. 1985. *Commodities and Capabilities*. Oxford: Oxford University Press.

———. 1999. *Development as Freedom*. New York: Knopf.

Spence, Michael, and Maureen Lewis. 2009. *Health and Growth*. Washington, DC: Commission on Growth and Development, World Bank.

Strauss, John, and Duncan Thomas. 2007. "Health over the Life Course." In *Handbook of Development*, vol. 4, edited by T. P. Schultz and J. Strauss. Amsterdam: North Holland Press.

Suhrcke, M., Regina Sauto Arce, Martin McKee, and Lorenzo Rocco. 2008. *The Economic Costs of Ill Health in the European Region*. Copenhagen: World Health Organization and the European Observatory on Health Systems and Policies.

Suhrcke, M., L. Rocco, and M. McKee. 2007. *Health: A Vital Investment for Economic Development in Eastern Europe and Central Asia*. Copenhagen: World Health Organization and the European Observatory on Health Systems and Policies.

Suhrcke, M., Lorenzo Rocco, Martin McKee, Stefano Mazzuco, Dieter Urban, and Alfred Steinherr. 2007. *Economics Consequences of Noncommunicable*

Diseases and Injuries in the Russian Federation. Copenhagen: World Health Organization and the European Observatory on Health Systems and Policies.

Victora, C. G., L. Adair, C. Fall, P. Hallal, R. Martorell, L. Richter, and H. Sachdev. 2008. "Maternal and Child Undernutrition: Consequences for Adult Health and Human Capital." *Lancet* 371: 340–57.

Viscusi, W. K. 1993. "The Value of Risks to Life and Health." *Journal of Economic Literature* 31 (4): 1912–46.

Viscusi, W. K., and J. Aldy. 2003. "The Value of a Statistical Life: A Critical Review of Market Estimates throughout the World." *Journal of Risk and Uncertainty* 27 (1): 5–76.

Weil, D. N. 2007. "Accounting for the Effect of Health on Economic Growth." *Quarterly Journal of Economics* 122 (3): 1265–1306.

World Bank. 1996. "Evaluating Public Spending: A Framework for Public Expenditure Reviews." Discussion Paper 323, World Bank, Washington, DC.

———. 2012. "Findings from a Household Survey On Health In 6 ECA Countries." Draft. World Bank, Washington, DC.

Yeh, Ethan. 2012. "Health and Income." Background report to *Getting Better*. World Bank, Washington, DC.

CHAPTER 3

Improving Health: The Heart of the Matter

Key Messages

- Cardiovascular disease, neonatal mortality, and injuries account for a very high percentage of the gap in life expectancy between ECA and the EU-15.

- A reduction in mortality due to cardiovascular disease and neonatal conditions has also been responsible for the majority of health gains in Western Europe over the past 50 years. Both prevention (especially smoking cessation) and treatment have been central to these successes.

- Smoking prevalence is notably higher in ECA than in the EU-15, especially among men. But a larger share of smokers in ECA is also trying to quit. In some countries, binge drinking is also more common.

- In most countries, there is widespread support for public health measures to help address tobacco and alcohol use; yet much can still be done to strengthen these policies. Public opinion is ahead of government action. Where measures have been taken, enforcement of existing regulations, especially those for alcohol, may be lacking.

- Women—who smoke and drink significantly less than men yet bear a disproportionate share of the consequences—are even more strongly in favor of stronger anti-tobacco and anti-alcohol policies than men. There is a strong gender dimension to these policy issues in ECA.

- In primary care, there are large gaps in the control of risk factors for cardiovascular disease, such as high blood pressure and cholesterol. Outpatient drug benefit packages to help treat these conditions should be improved, and strong disease management programs to guide the delivery of care should be established. Risk factor management should be measured, monitored, and possibly used as a basis for reimbursement.

- Between public health legislation and risk factor management through primary care, there are major health gains available for very low cost; the main gaps to be closed are not expensive. Most health improvement does not involve hospitals, which nevertheless gain undue attention and resources.

- The quality of care in ECA appears to be low in each of its three dimensions—structural, clinical processes, and patient outcomes—especially at the primary-care level. Effective interventions to improve quality of care should be systematically introduced and reinforced, especially those that aim to change provider behaviors through payment, professional recognition, and peer review.

The fundamental objective of a health system is to improve health outcomes, and this is the topic to which we now turn. As seen in chapter 1, the life expectancy gap between Europe and Central Asia (ECA) and the EU-15 has increased from 5 years to about 10 since the 1960s, in contrast to the global norm of narrowing health inequalities. This divergence is even sharper if Turkey is not included in the ECA average. What explains this gap, and how can it be closed? How to achieve more rapid convergence of health outcomes will guide the discussion in this chapter.

From the outset, it is important to note that there has been significant cross-country variation in health outcome trends within the region (see also box 1.1). Some countries, such as Turkey and the western Balkans, have made steady progress over the years in line with global experience. Others, such as those in Central Europe, had a long period of stagnation in the 1970s and 1980s but have since begun to catch up with Western Europe. Other new member states of the European Union (EU), including in southeastern Europe and the Baltics, have experienced more gradual improvements without closing the gap. There is also variation within the Commonwealth of Independent States (CIS), with some countries on a long plateau while others have had unprecedented fluctuations. Nevertheless, improving health outcomes is an ongoing challenge throughout the region, and thus the discussion that follows is relevant to all countries, even if not in equal measure.

The main outcome used in this report to highlight the challenge of improving health is life expectancy, a simple and well-known summary measure of population health. But it is less practical for monitoring the impact of specific policies and programs, for which more granular metrics are needed. In fact, developing a list of specific health outcome indicators and monitoring their trends over time are potentially key policy imperatives themselves. Some of the benchmarking of health indicators undertaken in this chapter can serve as a useful starting point in this respect.

While the focus here is mainly on health in ECA at the national level, most health indicators in the region vary by socioeconomic status, with the poor typically faring worse (Mackenbach et al. 2008; World Bank 2012b). A comprehensive health policy agenda would concern itself with not just the averages but also with the distribution of outcomes across society. While the question of how (or whether) to address income inequality directly is beyond the scope of this report, a key contribution that health systems can make in this regard is to strive for equal access to medical care regardless of socioeconomic status. This issue will be examined further in chapter 4.

The next section aims to highlight the importance of cardiovascular disease and a short list of other causes of death. The aim is not to promote more vertical programming, but rather to view the health convergence challenge through the lens of heart disease and then draw lessons for health systems more broadly. This approach is applied in three broad areas: public health, managing risk factors through primary care, and the quality of treatment and care. Throughout, extensive use is made of a tailored household survey implemented in six former Soviet republics (Azerbaijan, Georgia,

Moldova, the Russian Federation, Tajikistan, and Uzbekistan) using many of the same questions asked of households in 27 EU countries by *Eurobarometer*, thus enabling broad cross-country comparisons (European Commission, 2007, 2010).

The Main Source of the Life Expectancy Gap Is Cardiovascular Disease

What are the main determinants of individual and population health? There are many, of course. A list would have to include our genes, early childhood conditions, nutrition, knowledge about the factors that affect our health, educational level, personal behaviors (smoking, drinking, diet, exercise, safe sex, and the like), the environment (air and water quality), socioeconomic status, and medical care. All of these are likely to be relevant for ECA at least to some degree.

It is not possible to say exactly how much of a population's ill health is due to each of these underlying causes, in ECA or anywhere. There are too many interrelated factors and long time lags. For example, it is plausible that part of the life expectancy gap with the EU-15 is due to less favorable early childhood conditions in ECA during the 1920s and 1930s (Brainerd 2010; Kesternich et al. 2012). The complexity of "health production" poses a challenge for identifying policy priorities and measuring impact. But two lines of inquiry can go a long way toward establishing a preliminary diagnosis of what ails ECA and thus set the stage for the remainder of the chapter. The first is to account for the proximate determinants of mortality in the form of common measures of disease burden. The second is to look at the historical evidence on health improvements in countries with longer-living populations such as the EU-15 over the past 50 years, as that can be informative about what lies ahead for ECA. Both are discussed here.

A first step is to analyze mortality patterns. In keeping with the theme of convergence between Eastern and Western Europe, this analysis is presented as an age-, gender-, and cause-specific breakdown of the life expectancy gap between ECA and the EU-15. It has some similarities to other measures of avoidable mortality, such as "preventable deaths"—for example, if nobody smoked—or deaths that are "amenable to health care"—that is, if medical care were deployed to its maximum effect (Nolte and McKee 2003, 2004). But unlike those measures, the counterfactual here is real people and health systems in the EU-15, as opposed to "perfect" ones. Thus, it puts an emphasis on what is possible if ECA follows in the footsteps

FIGURE 3.1

Accounting for the Life Expectancy Gap between ECA and the EU-15

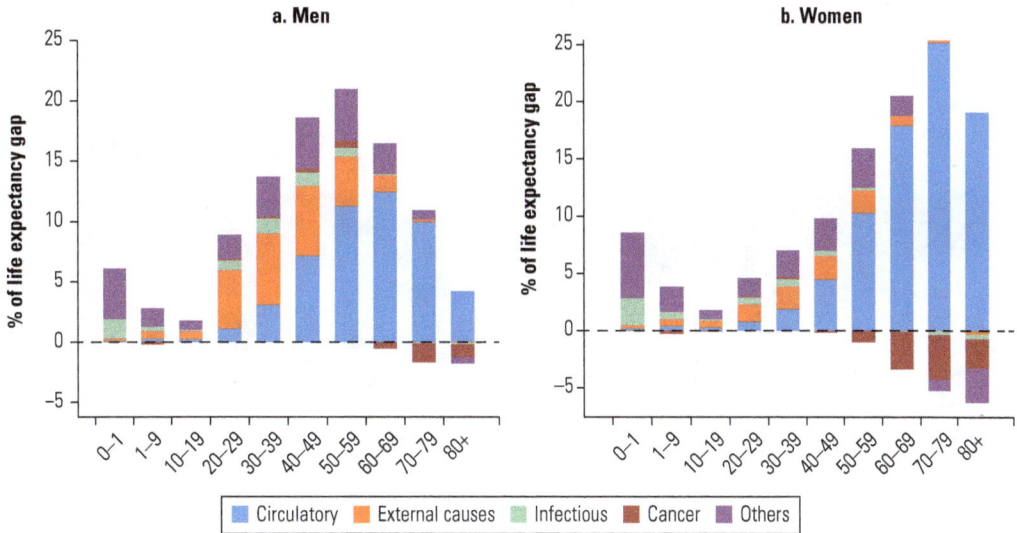

a. Men   b. Women

Source: Canudas-Romo 2011.
Note: ECA = Europe and Central Asia.

of that region's experience. The quality of cause-of-death data varies across ECA, but it is sufficient in most countries to yield robust policy messages.

Figure 3.1 shows the results of this exercise for ECA as a whole, undertaken as a background paper to this report (Canudas-Romo 2011). Three main findings stand out. First, across the region, the predominant source of the life expectancy gap is diseases of the circulatory system. These account for about half the gap among men and for more than 75 percent among women. The overwhelming importance of a single disease group, albeit a complex one, already sends a clear signal about ECA's lagging health outcomes and represents an obvious target for policy action. A second important reason for the longevity gap between ECA and the EU-15 is attributable to deaths before the age of one. Although fewer in number than other causes, these have a disproportionate effect on life expectancy. About two-thirds of infant mortality in ECA occurs during the neonatal period—that is, during the first 28 days (WHO 2010). A third key factor is external causes, most of which are attributable to road traffic injuries. These are most common among the male population, although women are also affected. Unlike the first two, this factor is most heavily concentrated in the working-age population.

The regionwide pattern masks some variation across countries. While the predominant role of cardiovascular disease is common

FIGURE 3.2

Accounting for the Life Expectancy Gain in the EU-15 for Males and Females, between 1965 and 2005

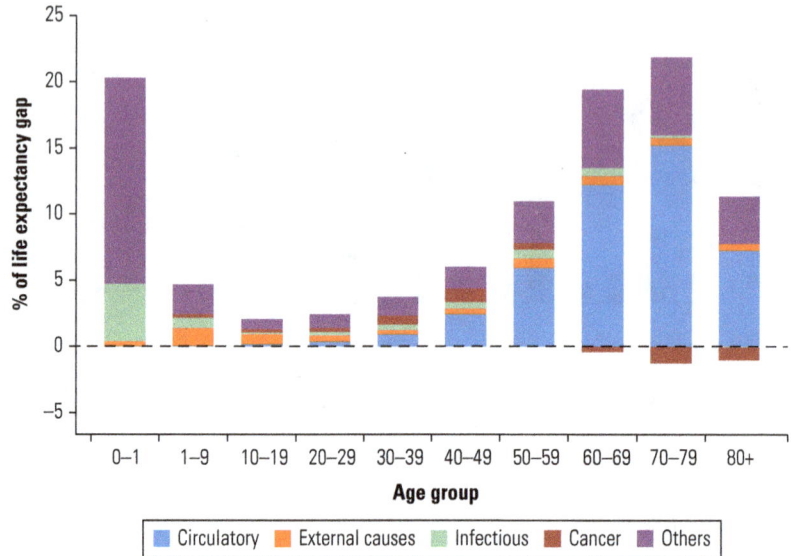

Source: Canudas-Romo 2011.

everywhere, the significance of infant deaths is more marked in Central Asia and the Caucasus. Also, the importance of external causes is most notable in Belarus, Kazakhstan, Russia, Ukraine, and the three Baltic nations. Elsewhere, they are not a major reason for the mortality gap.

The importance of cardiovascular and neonatal health can also be seen in the historical experience of the EU-15 over the past 50 years. Figure 3.2 decomposes the gain in life expectancy achieved in that region between 1965 and 2005. The decline in these two causes of death accounts for about two-thirds of the longevity gains for both men and women over this period. In the United States, reductions in mortality due to cardiovascular disease and deaths in infancy are estimated to have accounted for almost 90 percent of the gain in life expectancy between 1960 and 2000 (Cutler, Rosen, and Vijan 2006).

The central role of lower mortality from heart disease in extending life spans in the West over the past 50 years has been labeled the "cardiovascular revolution" (Vallin and Mesle 2001). It has arguably been the biggest success of modern medicine. In 1950, there was little that could be done to help a patient with heart disease, and knowledge of its causes was very incomplete. In 1964, the U.S. surgeon general issued a landmark report linking tobacco use with serious health consequences, helping shift public attitudes and trigger concerted policy action to reduce cigarette consumption. Knowledge and awareness of the links between heart health and diet, exercise, and alcohol intake have also improved significantly, although obesity rates have steadily increased in most rich countries since the 1970s (OECD 2011). Meanwhile, there have been enormous strides in pharmaceutical innovation and medical technology. Diuretics, beta-blockers, and ACE-inhibitors for hypertension; statins for cholesterol; and thrombolytics for heart attack and stroke have all had large impacts. Diagnostic techniques are also much better, and newly developed invasive procedures such as coronary artery bypass graft and angioplasty have made a difference as well, even if they are sometimes overused.

A number of studies have attempted to decompose the large reductions in cardiovascular disease in the West into its various causes (Tunstall-Pedoe et al. 2000; Nolte and McKee 2003; Cutler, Rosen, and Vijan 2006; Ford et al. 2007). This type of analysis is an inexact science, and the relative importance of the different factors is likely to vary by country and time period. But the exercise has important policy implications. A general rule of thumb is that prevention has contributed about 50 percent of the mortality reduction and treatment has been responsible for the other 50 percent. Some studies have attributed a larger role to treatment, others less. On the prevention side, the most important contributor has been tobacco cessation, while drugs have been the best treatment. But other factors have been important too. This track record suggests that neither prevention nor treatment alone will suffice to replicate the Western European experience in reducing deaths due to heart disease in ECA. Countries cannot prevent their way out of this disease burden, nor can medical care be relied upon to let people "off the hook" for their behavior. But it is also clear that the role of hospitals has been relatively small, with important implications for the efficiency of spending, as will be discussed in chapter 5.

An important caveat to the long-term mortality reduction that can be achieved by addressing cardiovascular disease *alone* arises from "competing risks." Everyone will die of one cause or another, and if deaths due to heart problems decrease, the risk of cancer, for example, will tend to increase in a partially offsetting way, especially in a population with a legacy of unhealthy behaviors. This factor helps shed light on why cancer rates in ECA are often lower than in the EU-15 (as indicated in figure 3.1), because people are dying of heart disease first. It also helps explain why cancer deaths rose as cardiovascular mortality fell in the West over a certain period, although in many cases, cancer rates are now falling, too. This topic will be revisited in a later section. But despite the reality of competing risks, the preeminence of cardiovascular disease, both as part of the problem and therefore as part of the solution, remains valid.

The second important contributor to the life expectancy gap shown in figure 3.1 is neonatal mortality. A similar story of remarkable progress exists for this aspect of the disease burden in Western Europe over the past several decades. Neonatal deaths in the EU-15 have fallen from about 20 per 1,000 in 1960 to less than 3 today (UNICEF 2010). In ECA today, the major direct causes of neonatal deaths are preterm complications, infections (especially pneumonia), and asphyxia, while low birthweight (less than 2,500 grams) is a major indirect cause (Black et al. 2010). The risk factors for low birthweight include harmful maternal behaviors such as smoking and excessive alcohol intake, as well as poor nutrition and maternal age. But it is notable that the prevalence of low birthweight is quite similar in ECA and the EU-15 and has not fallen by much in the latter region in recent decades. A large part of the difference lies in what happens in the first hours and days after birth. Neonatal care can achieve much more today than in the past. Where once the main option was an incubator, there are now ventilators and other new technologies for nourishing, monitoring, diagnosing, and treating low-birthweight infants. Perhaps even more than cardiovascular outcomes, medical care has played an important role in the reduction of neonatal mortality. In the future, the achievement of major reductions in neonatal deaths will depend on the provision of individualized clinical care (Lawn, Cousens, and Zupan 2005). As rates fall further, the role of technology (including expensive neonatal intensive-care units) will increase. The quality of neonatal care in ECA today is discussed in a later section.

The third major cause of the life expectancy gap—external causes—is different in the sense that it was never as high in the EU-15 as it is in ECA today and has not played such a large role in mortality reduction in the West. As noted, the problem is especially concentrated in seven countries in ECA. The most important subcategory is road traffic injuries, but others include homicide, suicide, poisonings, and others. Alcohol plays a central role in deaths due to external causes in ECA, and a policy agenda in this area is discussed in the next section since it is also a key risk factor for cardiovascular disease. Other policy levers for reducing this source of the disease burden include better road network planning, enforcement of safety laws (speeding, seat belts, helmets, and so forth), and emergency medical care (WHO 2004, 2009a).

In sum, this chapter will focus mostly on cardiovascular disease as the largest source of the life expectancy gap between ECA and the EU-15 and the major source of longevity gains in the West in the past 50 years. Both prevention and treatment have been, and will be, central to this story. The "disease-specific lens" afforded by cardiovascular disease will be used to draw out implications for ECA health systems in general along the way. Many of the key messages can be generalized to other conditions, since cardiovascular health requires a range of interventions from public health to the control of risk factors through primary care to more advanced treatments. Other key priorities include neonatal health, deaths due to external causes, and, eventually, cancer, and these will also be explored as appropriate. Analyzing health system performance at the disease level can shed more light on key challenges than highly aggregated studies (Garber 2003) and also provides an opportunity to identify actionable indicators for monitoring progress.

While this chapter focuses on cardiovascular disease, there is an unfinished agenda related to the Millennium Development Goals (MDGs). Three of the eight MDGs pertain directly to health—reducing child mortality, improving maternal health, and combating HIV/AIDS and tuberculosis. Specific targets include reducing the under-five mortality rate by two-thirds between 1990 and 2015, lowering the maternal mortality ratio by three-quarters over the same period, and beginning to reduce the spread of HIV/AIDS by 2015. Strictly interpreted, many countries in ECA have not achieved these targets, in part because their 1990 baseline values were generally better than in most other developing countries; they had reached a point at which incremental changes had become increasingly difficult to achieve. Due to the predominance of noncommunicable diseases in ECA's disease burden, some have questioned the appropriateness of the MDGs for the region (Rechel, Shapo, and McKee 2005).

The monitoring of progress toward the MDGs has focused on 75 "countdown countries" with higher burdens, of which five are in ECA: Azerbaijan, the Kyrgyz Republic, Tajikistan, Turkmenistan, and Uzbekistan. As of 2010, most had made progress in reducing child and maternal mortality, but the MDG targets remain elusive (Countdown 2012). Most child mortality in ECA is during the neonatal period (first 28 days). Maternal mortality is fortunately a rare event in ECA. As of 2008, there were fewer than 2,000 maternal deaths across the region (about the same as in Brazil), and 20 countries in the region had fewer than 25 annually nationwide. But it remains an important challenge in some countries, particularly in Central Asia.

Box 3.1 provides a brief overview of the challenges that ECA is facing in addressing HIV/AIDS and tuberculosis.

An Unfinished Agenda: HIV/AIDS and Tuberculosis in ECA

There were around 1.5 million people living with HIV/AIDS in ECA at the end of 2010. Since 2001, HIV prevalence in ECA has increased by 250 percent, in contrast to declining or stabilizing HIV epidemics elsewhere in the world. ECA, therefore, has the fastest-growing epidemic in the world, although its prevalence rate (0.9 percent) is still much lower than that of Sub-Saharan Africa (5 percent). Russia and Ukraine account for almost 90 percent of ECA's reported new infections.

The HIV epidemic in ECA is driven primarily by the practice of sharing equipment among injecting drug users (IDUs) and sexual transmission from infected IDUs to their sex partners. IDUs constitute around 59 percent of the total number of HIV/AIDS cases in ECA. Around one-quarter of the estimated 3.7 million IDUs in the region are living with the disease. Among 1.8 million IDUs in Russia, this rate is 37 percent. However, the coverage of evidence-based, cost-effective HIV interventions for IDUs such as needle and syringe programs and opiate substitution therapy is inadequate. No ECA country has been able to reach the coverage levels of needle and syringe programs and opiate substitution therapy recommended by the World Health Organization (WHO). Opiate substitution therapy is not offered in Russia.

Voluntary counseling and testing, another key HIV intervention, remain limited for at-risk groups such as IDUs, sex workers, and men who have sex with men in ECA. In countries for which data were available in 2009, none has achieved more than 50 percent coverage of voluntary counseling and testing among these populations. With regard to treatment, only 23 percent of those in need of anti-retroviral therapy in ECA currently receive it, which is less than half the treatment coverage rate in Sub-Saharan Africa. Provision of anti-retroviral therapy in ECA is the second lowest of any region (only the Middle East and North Africa is lower) and is not keeping pace with new infections. While IDUs comprise the majority of people living with HIV/AIDS, they represent less than a quarter of those currently under treatment. In general, at-risk populations are neglected in government allocations to HIV/AIDS programs and are instead covered largely by international funding sources (UNGASS 2010; UNAIDS 2012; UNECE 2012).

To effectively address the HIV/AIDS challenge, ECA countries need to do the following: (1) scale up needle and syringe programs and opiate substitution therapy interventions for IDUs; (2) expand voluntary counseling and testing for the most at-risk groups such as IDUs, commercial sex workers, and men who have sex with men; and (3) widen access to anti-retroviral therapy. Achievements of such goals would require, among other things: (1) increasing resource allocations for effective, evidence-based interventions targeting at-risk groups; (2) improving programming and implementation of such interventions in partnership with civil society; and (3) removing punitive laws where they exist, as they are obstacles to access to prevention, treatment, care, and support by the most at-risk populations.

continued

BOX 3.1 *continued*

Tuberculosis (TB), a disease strongly linked to poverty, remains a key health risk in ECA, where it is a topic of global importance. While new EU member states have made gains against TB since its peak in the late 1990s, the opposite is true in CIS countries, where progress in TB control during the Soviet era has been reversed. TB incidence has doubled since 1990 in CIS countries, and it is now almost three times higher than among new EU member states and ten times higher than in Western Europe. As a result, attaining the MDG for tuberculosis in these countries is not on track. ECA also has some of the worst TB treatment outcomes in the world, with a success rate of 65 percent, and the spread of drug-resistant tuberculosis is on the rise. The region has the highest rates of multi-drug-resistant TB in the world, with 32 percent of new cases and 76 percent of previously treated cases resistant to at least two of the most potent TB drugs. The number of TB deaths has doubled in ECA during the past 20 years, particularly among working-age men. The policy imperative is to improve case detection rates and treatment outcomes and aggressively address TB-HIV co-infections.

Smoking, Drinking, Men, and Women: More Can Be Done to Address Tobacco and Alcohol Use

The starting point for reducing mortality from cardiovascular disease is to address its major risk factors in the general population before individuals need medical care. The focus here is on two of the most important, tobacco and alcohol use. Cigarette smoking damages the blood vessels, impedes the transfer of oxygen from the lungs, and puts the heart under increased strain. Excessive alcohol consumption raises blood pressure, leads to damage of the coronary arteries, and can directly affect the heart muscle. Both raise the risk of heart attack and stroke, among other dangers (which also include cancer). Smokers live about seven years less than nonsmokers. There is also a link between smoking and drinking during pregnancy and the probability of low-birthweight infants, posing a risk to neonatal health, and alcohol contributes to road traffic deaths. Thus, tobacco and alcohol matter for many reasons.

Behavior change is one of the most difficult tasks for government policy to accomplish. Who partakes in unhealthy behaviors, and why they do so, can be quite idiosyncratic and strongly influenced by social factors and individual circumstance. At the country level, different nations have both their virtues and vices. Within the Organisation for Economic Co-operation and Development (OECD), the United States has the highest rate of obesity but one of the lowest rates of tobacco use; Greece has the highest rate of tobacco use and the lowest suicide rate; France has the highest rate of alcohol consumption and one of the lowest obesity rates. The same is true of individuals. In six ECA countries surveyed, there was very little correlation between whether a survey respondent was a smoker, was a binge drinker, was obese, wore a seat belt in a car, or had a physical checkup in the past year. The same has been observed in other countries. The challenge is to change the action, not the person. The difficulty of doing so should not be underestimated, but there are also effective policies available.

This section compares ECA with the EU-15 on the prevalence of smoking and excessive drinking, knowledge about their health effects, public attitudes toward potential policy measures, and current policy efforts to address these problems. Other cardiovascular risk factors, such as diet and exercise, and the broader public health agenda are noted briefly at the end.

A Smoke-Filled Region

People smoke more in ECA than in almost any other region. The prevalence, frequency, and intensity of cigarette use by males in 18 ECA countries with data comparable to the EU-15 are shown in figure 3.3. About one-third of men in the EU-15 classify themselves as current smokers, a rate that is exceeded, often by a wide margin, in the majority of ECA countries. Over 90 percent of smokers in ECA light up on a daily basis, compared with less than three-quarters in the EU-15, and most of them also smoke more cigarettes per day. ECA is also a region of heavy tobacco use by global standards. New research on smoking prevalence in 14 large middle-income countries representing 3 billion people found that Russia, Turkey, and Ukraine had the three highest rates of smoking prevalence of males between the ages of 15 and 34 (Giovino et al. 2012). Smoking among youth is an ill omen for future health.

The prevalence of smoking among women in ECA is notably lower than among men, ranging from below 5 percent in Central Asia and the Caucasus to over 20 percent in the EU-15 and most of the new EU member states in ECA. The gender disparity in tobacco use is a major reason for the significant gap in life expectancy between men and women in the region. But while women smoke less than men, the gap may be narrowing. There is evidence comparing eight former Soviet countries in 2001 and 2010 that suggests that men are smoking somewhat less than previously but that women are smoking slightly more (Roberts et al. 2012).

FIGURE 3.3

Men in ECA Smoke More than Men in the EU-15

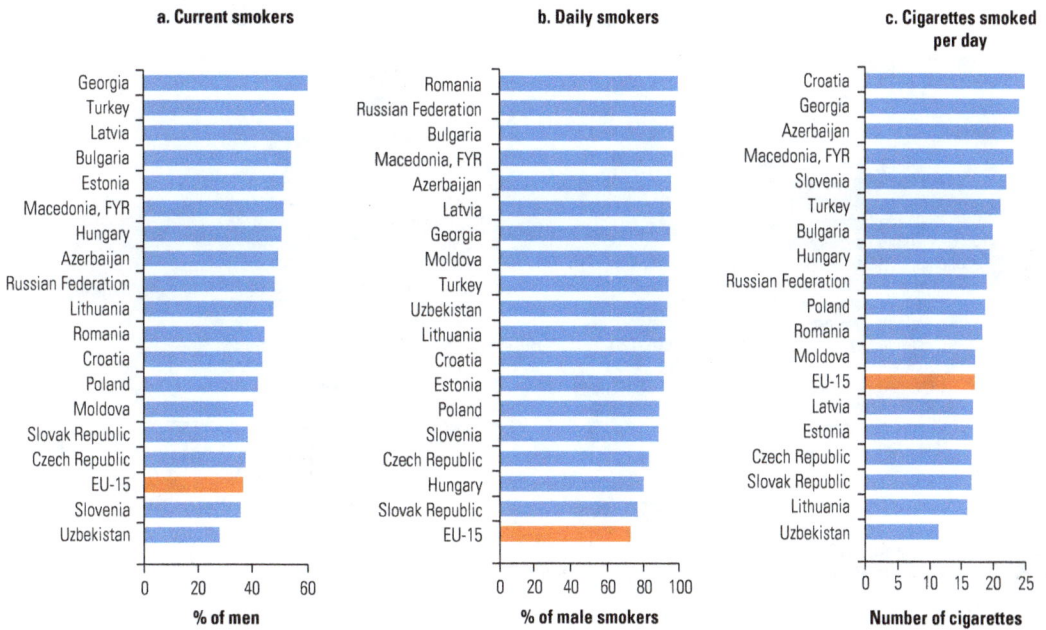

a. Current smokers
% of men

Georgia
Turkey
Latvia
Bulgaria
Estonia
Macedonia, FYR
Hungary
Azerbaijan
Russian Federation
Lithuania
Romania
Croatia
Poland
Moldova
Slovak Republic
Czech Republic
EU-15
Slovenia
Uzbekistan

b. Daily smokers
% of male smokers

Romania
Russian Federation
Bulgaria
Macedonia, FYR
Azerbaijan
Latvia
Georgia
Moldova
Turkey
Uzbekistan
Lithuania
Croatia
Estonia
Poland
Slovenia
Czech Republic
Hungary
Slovak Republic
EU-15

c. Cigarettes smoked per day
Number of cigarettes

Croatia
Georgia
Azerbaijan
Macedonia, FYR
Slovenia
Turkey
Bulgaria
Hungary
Russian Federation
Poland
Romania
Moldova
EU-15
Latvia
Estonia
Czech Republic
Slovak Republic
Lithuania
Uzbekistan

Sources: European Commission 2010; World Bank 2012a.
Note: ECA = Europe and Central Asia.

Smoking is commonplace in ECA, but what is the role of public policy in addressing individual choices related to tobacco use? It is sometimes argued that if people want to smoke, governments should not make it their business to stop them. The most obvious reason is the externality of second-hand smoke, which poses health risks to others in public places but especially within households. In ECA countries with higher tobacco use, about one-quarter of survey respondents state that they are "very often" bothered by exposure to smoke in their daily lives, about twice as high as in most of the EU-15. Smoking is also expensive and can crowd out household spending on other items, including food and human capital investments such as health and education, especially among low-income families (Wang, Sindelar, and Busch 2006). In many ECA countries, smoking prevalence is similar across socioeconomic quintiles, and thus tobacco accounts for a larger share of household spending among the poor.

Policies to address tobacco use have also been justified on the grounds that most smokers want to quit. In six former Soviet countries where the question was asked, about two-thirds of smokers said they would like to quit. In most ECA countries, between one-quarter

FIGURE 3.4

Smokers Are Trying to Kick the Habit, but Often Not Succeeding

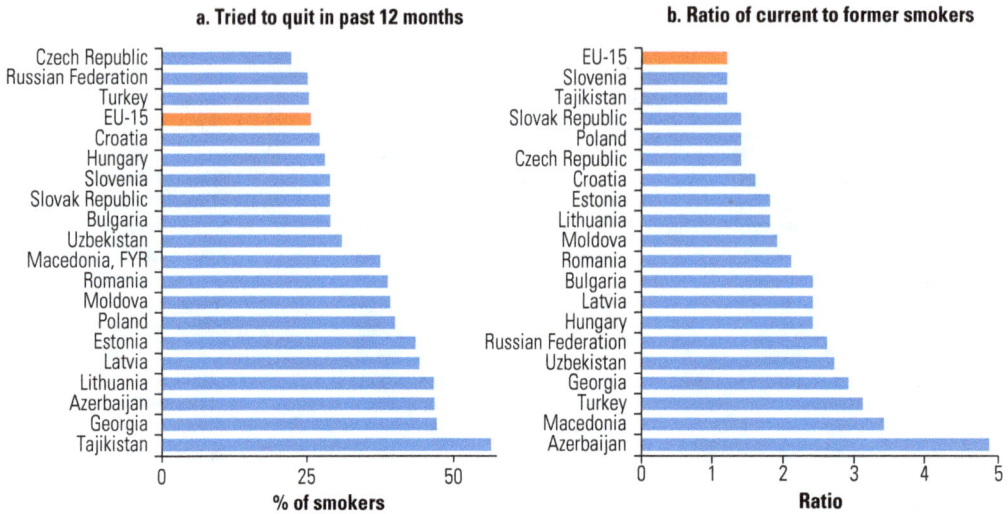

a. Tried to quit in past 12 months

b. Ratio of current to former smokers

Sources: European Commission 2010; World Bank 2012a.
Note: Figure shows data for countries in Europe and Central Asia and the EU-15.

and one-half of smokers report that they have tried to quit during the past 12 months, a higher share than in the EU-15 (figure 3.4). But quitting is hard. The average age at which male smokers in ECA began their habit is just 17, and addiction takes hold quickly. The success rate of ECA's smokers who are trying to quit is lower than in the EU-15, as indicated by the ratio of current to former smokers (figure 3.4). This difference is partly a reflection of a less supportive policy environment for would-be quitters, as discussed below. These survey responses provide support to the behavioral economics theory that tobacco use reflects a problem of time-inconsistent preferences—that is, people want to quit tomorrow but not today—more than so-called "rational addiction" in which people want to smoke despite the risks (Gruber and Koszegi 2001). The implication is that optimal policy making could make people better off by helping address the problem whereby a person's behavior today may inflict costs on their "future self" down the road.

About three-quarters or more of ECA's smokers who report that they tried to quit during the past year cited personal health as a motivating factor, in addition to other reasons such as the cost of smoking. This finding suggests that ECA's smokers are well aware of the health consequences of their habit. In fact, there is little difference with the EU-15 in this respect. Over 80 percent of survey respondents in six former Soviet countries agree with the statement that "smoking causes cancer and death," a rate similar to the EU-15. A large majority of respondents in 16 ECA countries surveyed on the matter also recognize the potential health consequences of second-hand smoke, again similar to the EU-15. Thus, a lack of awareness of the health consequences of smoking does not appear to be a major reason for high tobacco use in ECA.

Policy levers for reducing tobacco use include cigarette taxation, smoking bans in public places such as offices and restaurants, restrictions on advertising tobacco products and sales to youth, warning labels on packages, nicotine replacement therapies to help those trying to quit, and general medical advice through primary care. A comprehensive review of national anti-tobacco policies suggests that on many of these fronts, countries in ECA are doing less than countries in Western Europe (WHO 2011a).

The most effective anti-tobacco policy is to increase cigarette taxes. In fact, it has been identified as one of the most cost-effective of all health interventions (Laxminarayan et al. 2006). A large research literature suggests that a 10 percent increase in cigarette prices will reduce overall consumption by about 2.5 to 5 percent in high-income countries, and the same price increase will have an even larger impact in low- or middle-income settings (Chaloupka et al. 2010; Cawley and Ruhm 2012). Over two-thirds of smokers in ECA say that price affects their choice of cigarette, compared to less than half in the EU-15. The responsiveness of cigarette consumption to price is also higher among youth, especially in lower-income settings (Kostova et al. 2010), and thus tobacco taxation can play a key role in deterring uptake in the first place. Since cigarette consumption typically falls by less than the price increase (that is, it is relatively price inelastic), the evidence on tobacco taxation also shows that higher taxes increase tax revenues, which should help allay concerns of treasury officials. Concerted multilateral efforts on tobacco taxation can also help confront the possible emergence of a smuggling problem. It should be acknowledged, however, that taxing cigarettes can be regressive.

Despite the strong supporting evidence in favor of higher tobacco taxation, there is substantial room for further increases in many countries in ECA and especially in the CIS region (figure 3.5). All EU countries have cigarette taxes that exceed 75 percent of the retail prices, while most Balkan countries fall just short of this level. But most CIS countries are well below 50 percent.

Another area in which ECA's anti-tobacco policies lag behind the EU-15's is the implementation of smoking bans in public

Tobacco Taxation Can Be Strengthened in Many ECA Countries

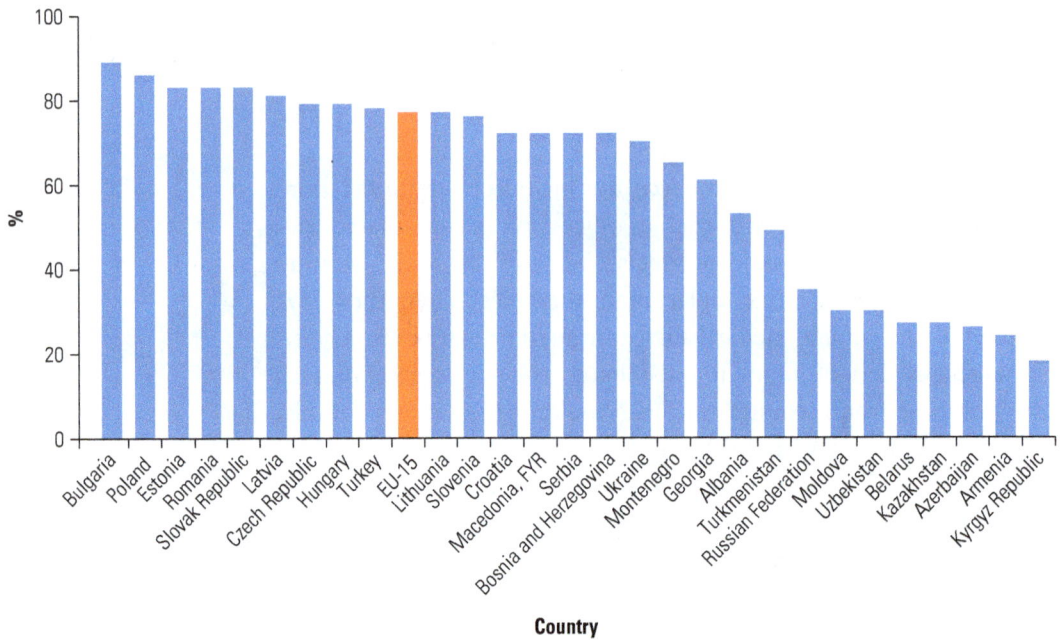

Source: WHO 2011a.
Note: Figure shows cigarette taxes as a percentage of the 2011 retail price. ECA = Europe and Central Asia.

places. In recent years, there has been a growing trend to enact legislation on this issue, beginning with Ireland in 2004 and spreading rapidly across much of the Continent (EPHA 2012). Enforcement is not always complete, but the trend has been both successful and broadly popular (Spinney 2007). But farther east, public smoking bans are less common (WHO 2011a), although in early 2013, Russia approved tough new anti-tobacco legislation. By taxing cigarettes at a higher rate and imposing public smoking bans, among other measures, governments could help "nudge" smokers into quitting and thus achieve more favorable ratios than those shown in figure 3.4.

The Gender Divide

Popular opinion is also in favor of stronger anti-tobacco policies, especially among women (figure 3.6). Both higher cigarette taxes and smoking bans in restaurants have the support of a majority of survey respondents across the region. There is little difference between ECA and the EU-15 on this front. In most countries, there is

FIGURE 3.6

There Is Widespread Support in ECA and the EU-15 for Anti-Tobacco Measures, Especially among Women

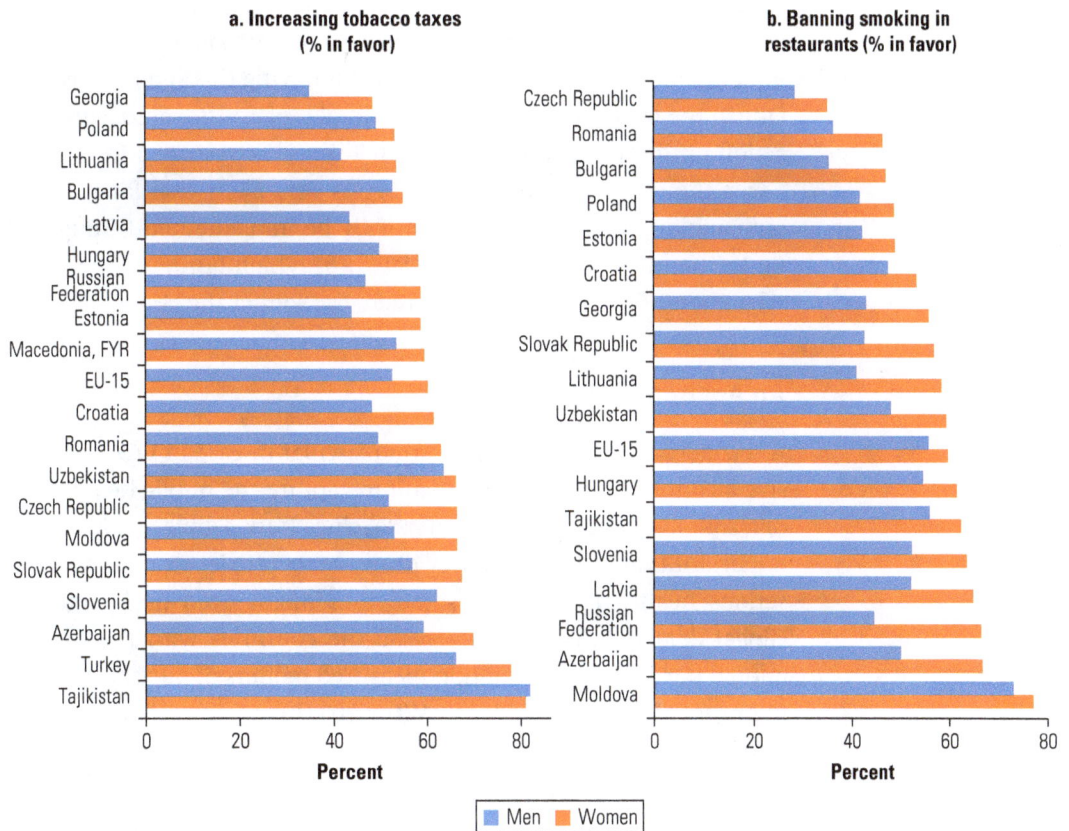

a. Increasing tobacco taxes (% in favor)

Countries (top to bottom): Georgia, Poland, Lithuania, Bulgaria, Latvia, Hungary, Russian Federation, Estonia, Macedonia, FYR, EU-15, Croatia, Romania, Uzbekistan, Czech Republic, Moldova, Slovak Republic, Slovenia, Azerbaijan, Turkey, Tajikistan

b. Banning smoking in restaurants (% in favor)

Countries (top to bottom): Czech Republic, Romania, Bulgaria, Poland, Estonia, Croatia, Georgia, Slovak Republic, Lithuania, Uzbekistan, EU-15, Hungary, Tajikistan, Slovenia, Latvia, Russian Federation, Azerbaijan, Moldova

Legend: Men, Women

Sources: European Commission 2007, 2010; World Bank 2012a.
Note: ECA = Europe and Central Asia.

a roughly 10-percentage-point gap between male and female support for these measures, with women more in favor.

The anti-tobacco agenda has a strong gender dimension in ECA. Smoking prevalence is far higher among men, representing a drain on household resources at the expense of women, inflicting second-hand smoke on those living under the same roof, and contributing to the large life expectancy gap between genders in the region (and thus widespread widowhood). One of the most comprehensive analyses of the cost of smoking identifies the impact on household members as the most significant external cost of tobacco use (Sloan et al. 2004). In ECA, this typically means men imposing a burden on women. This factor may help explain the gender gap in attitudes toward anti-tobacco legislation shown in figure 3.6, although it should be noted that in many countries a majority of men also support these measures.

In sum, there is an outstanding policy agenda for addressing high rates of smoking in ECA. Significantly, the most effective measures would come at very little budgetary cost and could in fact raise revenues. In general, public support for these steps is well in front of government action, suggesting a need for policy makers to play catch-up. Leadership will assume a key role in moving this agenda forward. One of the most successful recent examples of anti-tobacco legislative action in the region can be found in Turkey, as described in box 3.2. Given the experience of the EU-15, it is very likely that far-reaching anti-smoking measures will eventually be implemented throughout ECA. The question is when. In view of the high burden imposed by tobacco in ECA, especially on women, the sooner the better.

An Agenda for Alcohol

A second major risk factor for cardiovascular disease in ECA is excessive alcohol use. It is more difficult to capture the public health risks of alcohol in basic consumption data, since how people drink is more important than how much they drink. Moderate levels do not pose a serious health risk (and in some cases might even be beneficial). Global data indicate that nearly all the countries with the highest annual per capita consumption measured in liters of pure alcohol are in Europe, both East and West (WHO 2011b).

A more informative measure of the health risks related to alcohol is the frequency of so-called heavy episodic or binge drinking. Various definitions exist, making data comparisons difficult (WHO 2012a). One definition is five or more drinks in one sitting, for which figure 3.7 shows comparative data across the region. Binge drinking among men is more common in several ECA countries than in the EU-15, especially in the Baltic republics and Russia. In all countries, binge drinking among women is far less common. The very high result for Georgia reflects a tradition of wine drinking at feasts. Other countries with heavy episodic drinking for which comparable data are not available include Belarus, Kazakhstan, and Ukraine. In general, the significance of excessive alcohol consumption as a key driver of the life expectancy gap between ECA and the EU-15 is concentrated in fewer countries than in the case of tobacco.

The public health consequences of excessive drinking appear to be widely recognized across the region. Figure 3.8 indicates that respondents in every ECA country surveyed are more likely to agree that a person should not drive after consuming one drink compared to the EU-15. In nearly every country, they are also more likely to "totally agree" that alcohol can increase the risk of heart disease. A similar

BOX 3.2

A Strong Policy Response for Tobacco Control in Turkey

Smoking has long been a deeply rooted tradition in Turkey, especially among males. Between 1980 and 2000, tobacco use in Turkey nearly doubled, with annual cigarette sales increasing from US$55 billion to US$100 billion. There are currently about 16 million adult smokers in Turkey, and it has the highest male smoking rate among OECD countries at about 50 percent. Among women, around 15 percent are smokers, and this rate is on the rise. Over 50,000 people die each year from tobacco-related diseases, and among men, they are the most common cause of death. Without effective tobacco control measures, it has been estimated that the number of annual tobacco-attributable deaths would reach 127,000 by 2050. Until recently, Turkey was also one of the major tobacco-producing countries in the world.

Turkey's first tobacco control law was passed in 1996, and in 2004, the Turkish Parliament ratified the Framework Convention on Tobacco Control, an international treaty to reduce tobacco consumption under the auspices of WHO. In recent years, the government has stepped up its commitment to curbing the smoking epidemic. In 2008 and 2012, further amendments to tobacco control legislation were passed. As a result, Turkey now has some of the most comprehensive and advanced tobacco control measures in the world. These include:

- An increase in the tobacco tax to about 75 percent of the retail price

- A complete ban on smoking in public places, on advertising and promotion of tobacco products, and on sales of tobacco products to minors

- Prominent picture-based health warnings

- Generic packaging of cigarettes

- Public anti-smoking campaigns

- Increased access to smoking cessation products and treatment

In 2010, Turkey ranked fourth in the European Tobacco Control Scale published by the Association of European Cancer Leagues. Although existing prevalence data may not yet capture the impact of these recent measures, emerging evidence points to positive results from Turkey's advanced tobacco control program. Since the implementation of the expanded smoke-free law in 2008 and the tax increase in January 2010, cigarette sales in Turkey have decreased by 10.7 percent.

In addition to the government's high level of commitment, the success of tobacco control in Turkey can also be attributed to very good multisectoral collaboration and a strong civil society movement for tobacco control. More than 100 government agencies and nongovernmental organizations participated in the preparation of the National Tobacco Control Program and Plan of Action in 2008. The Turkish National Coalition on Tobacco or Health consists of more than 40 Turkish organizations working on tobacco control. The coalition has been very active in advocating for stringent and comprehensive tobacco control laws and monitoring the reinforcement of such laws.

FIGURE 3.7

There Is More Binge Drinking in Some ECA Countries

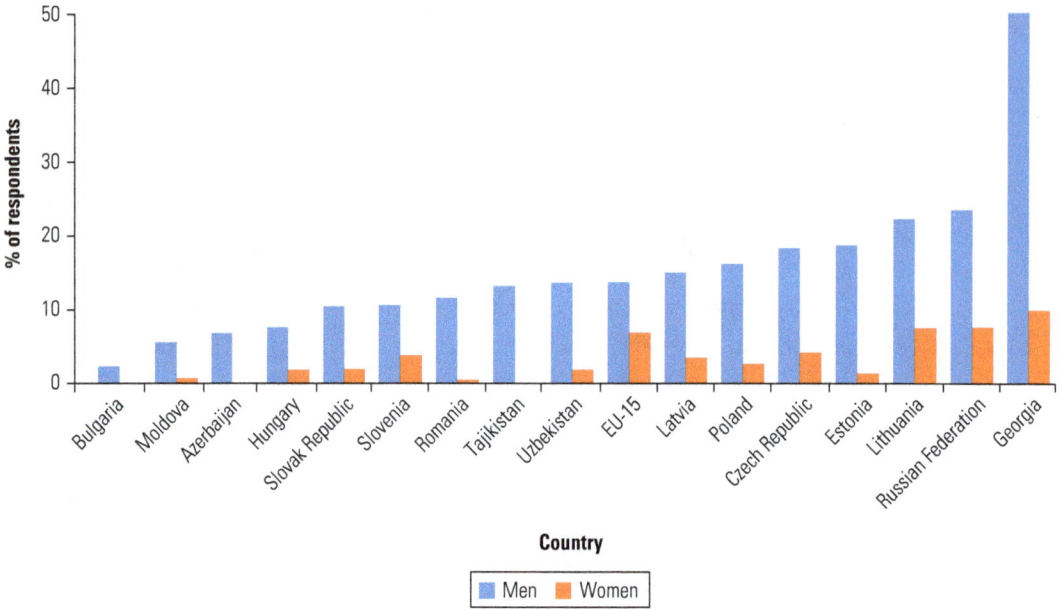

Sources: European Commission 2010; World Bank 2012a.
Note: Figure shows the consumption of five or more drinks in one sitting. ECA = Europe and Central Asia.

FIGURE 3.8

There Is Strong Knowledge of the Risks and Consequences of Alcohol Use in ECA

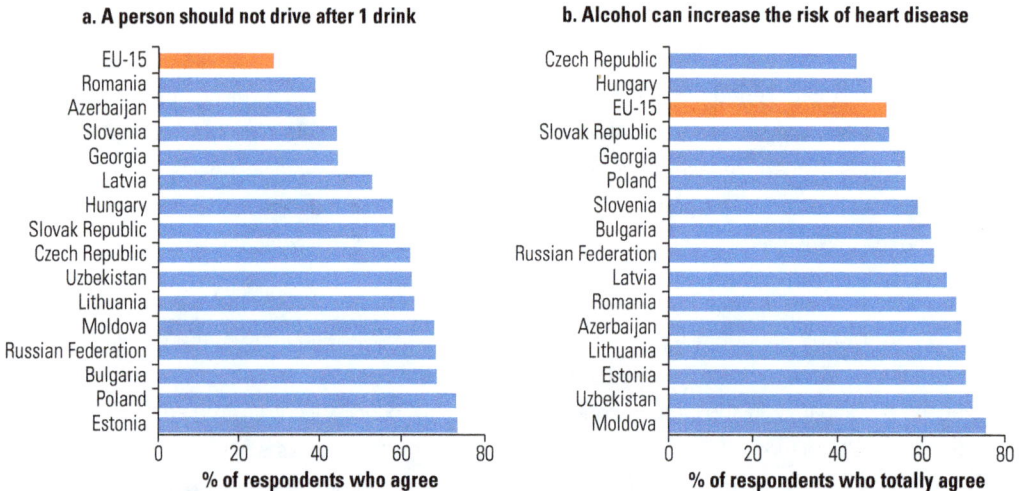

Sources: European Commission 2010; World Bank 2012a.
Note: ECA = Europe and Central Asia.

pattern prevails when they are asked about other health risks associated with alcohol, such as liver disease, depression, and birth defects. In addition, roughly half of binge drinkers in six ECA countries acknowledge that they need to reduce their drinking. While ongoing public awareness efforts are important, as with tobacco use, knowledge of the risks does not appear to be the major barrier to addressing the challenge of excessive alcohol consumption in ECA.

As with smoking, there are substantial external costs associated with excessive alcohol use that lend support to policy interventions. The extraordinary loss of life in ECA due to injuries as shown in figure 3.1, mainly concentrated during middle age, provides strong evidence of these costs. But because moderate, responsible alcohol consumption is not harmful, policy instruments such as taxation can be blunt tools. A large research literature has examined the price responsiveness of alcohol use, with results similar to that of tobacco (that is, elasticity near −0.5). However, heavy drinkers may be less responsive to higher prices (Cawley and Ruhm 2012).

In addition to taxation, policy options for addressing excessive alcohol use include warning labels, limiting its availability (for example, to youth or the hours of sale), enforcement of laws to reduce drinking and driving, advertising restrictions, awareness campaigns, and advice and treatment through the health system to help those in need. A stock taking of national policies reveals a mixed picture (WHO 2011b). For example, most ECA countries have more restrictive laws applied to limits on blood alcohol content when driving than the EU-15. Sales to youth are restricted nearly everywhere, and most countries have some advertising restrictions. But there is less comparable information available on alcohol taxation.

There is broader popular support in ECA than in the EU-15 for many anti-alcohol measures, such as warning labels and restricting access for youth. As in the case of tobacco, these policies are also more widely supported among women (who partake less in alcohol consumption) than men, although again a majority of the latter also supports them. Women are also more likely to agree that public authorities should intervene to protect people from alcohol-related harm, rather than saying that individuals are responsible enough to protect themselves.

In brief, there are many similarities between the alcohol agenda discussed here and the tobacco issues noted above. These behaviors are more prevalent in ECA than in the EU-15 and more common among men than women, while knowledge of the health risks is strong and popular support for public health measures to address excessive consumption is widespread. Policy measures for addressing

BOX 3.3

Addressing the Challenge of Alcohol Consumption in Russia

The challenge of addressing alcohol use in Russia goes back several decades (Stickley, Razvodovsky, and McKee 2009), but consumption started to increase more sharply after 1970. In recognition of the problem, a series of sweeping reforms was introduced to curtail alcohol consumption in the Soviet Union beginning in 1985. These included a sharp reduction in state production of alcohol, sales restrictions, price increases, and improved health education and treatment programs. Together, these steps were very successful at reducing alcohol-related mortality during the late 1980s. But the breakdown of these measures as a result of the dissolution of the Soviet Union is responsible for up to half the mortality spike in the early 1990s (Bhattacharya, Gathmann, and Miller, forthcoming). The sharp decline in the price of vodka in the early 1990s, corresponding to the breakdown of Gorbachev-era controls, was a major reason for the increased mortality at that time (Treisman 2010). This experience underlines the significance of the price channel in affecting alcohol use and therefore the promise of taxation as a policy instrument. More broadly, an array of policies can be used to help address alcohol use in Russia (World Bank 2005). The challenge of addressing excessive alcohol consumption in Russia is ongoing (Leon, Shkolnikov, and McKee 2009). In 2011, a law was signed to raise alcohol taxes significantly over the period 2012–14. Stronger enforcement of existing legislation and innovative public health campaigns to help shift attitudes will also be important.

alcohol could be strengthened, but, perhaps equally important, existing measures could also be better enforced. The successful anti-alcohol measures introduced in the Soviet Union during the late 1980s are discussed in box 3.3.

The Broader Public Health Agenda

Tobacco and alcohol are not the only risk factors for cardiovascular disease. Among others, diet and exercise are also important, but cross-country data for assessing differences are less readily available. Obesity rates, defined as a body mass index over 30, vary widely within both ECA and the EU-15 (OECD 2010), although overall they would appear to be higher in ECA. In both Eastern and Western Europe, the long-term trend has been an increase in the prevalence of obesity over time. Thus, the EU-15 has made significant progress against cardiovascular disease mortality despite rising obesity, although the delayed effect on the disease burden has probably yet to emerge fully. Policies to help address obesity may include food regulation and possibly taxation, although these are also in their infancy in more advanced health systems. In brief, the evidence base and rationale for intervening are somewhat less clear than for tobacco and alcohol.

A strengthening of public health measures to reduce cardiovascular disease can also serve as a springboard to undertaking deeper reforms in public health systems that have traditionally focused on other areas such as communicable disease and environmental health (Gotsadze et al. 2010). A greater focus on prevention of noncommunicable disease will be essential to managing the main source of ECA's disease burden. More generally, the public health agenda would benefit from strong leadership, a key ingredient in helping align government action closer to popular opinion on key public health issues, including tobacco and alcohol use.

There Are Big Gaps in Managing Risk Factors through Primary Care

The population-based interventions of the previous section can play a key role in preventing the emergence of cardiovascular disease, and they can be reinforced by health workers who advise and assist patients in addressing issues related to tobacco, alcohol, diet, and exercise. But inevitably there will be people with risk factors who come into contact with the medical care system, many of whom can be successfully treated through primary care. In that way, they can also be kept out of hospitals. This section examines how well countries in ECA are doing in this respect.

Taking the Pulse of Primary Care

High blood pressure, or hypertension, is the most important health risk factor both in ECA and in the world when measured by attributable mortality, far ahead of the second most important, tobacco use. About 30 percent of deaths in ECA can be attributed to hypertension (WHO 2009b). High cholesterol is also among the top-five risk factors. As noted earlier, better control of hypertension and cholesterol—in part through anti-hypertensive drugs and statins, respectively—has played a major role in the "cardiovascular revolution" achieved in the West in recent decades.

On the surface, ECA has made some effort to address heart health. When asked whether they have had a heart checkup and a blood pressure test during the previous 12 months, survey respondents in ECA were often at least as likely to say yes as those in the EU-15 (figure 3.9). More generally, outpatient health visits per capita in

FIGURE 3.9
Some Positive Signs in Cardiovascular Risk Management in ECA

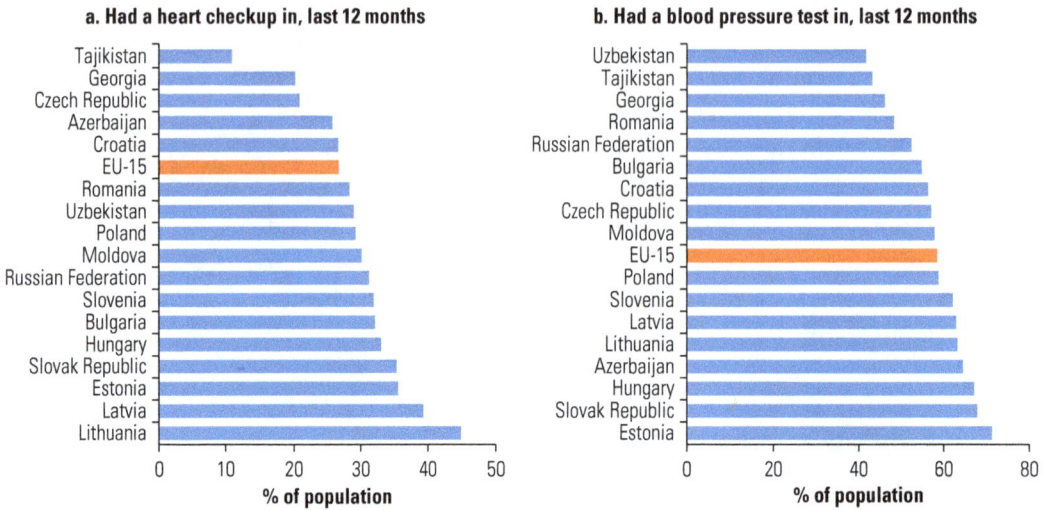

a. Had a heart checkup in, last 12 months

b. Had a blood pressure test in, last 12 months

Sources: European Commission 2007; World Bank 2012a.
Note: ECA = Europe and Central Asia.

ECA are slightly higher than in the EU-15, although there is significant country variation (WHO 2012b). But it is less clear what exactly these visits entail. A brief exam with a stethoscope or blood pressure meter will not translate into better health outcomes without follow-up by both doctor and patient.

The picture is less favorable if the focus is shifted to hypertension awareness, treatment, and control. Awareness rates refer to the share of those with high blood pressure who know that they have the condition. Treatment rates represent the share of those with hypertension who are taking medication. Control rates reflect a blood pressure reading below 140/90 among those on treatment as a share of all those with hypertension. In survey work undertaken as background to this report, blood pressure measurements were taken for over 6,000 respondents across six former Soviet republics, and the results were compared to recent nationally representative estimates in the medical literature for several other countries in ECA and some advanced systems. As indicated in figure 3.10, ECA lags behind at each link in the chain, culminating in control rates of roughly 10 percent in most ECA countries, compared to 30–60 percent in available comparators in Canada, the United Kingdom, and the United States. In the six former Soviet republics, blood pressure control rates among women were significantly better than among men. More generally, utilization rates of outpatient care across ECA are higher among women.

FIGURE 3.10

High Blood Pressure Is Not under Control

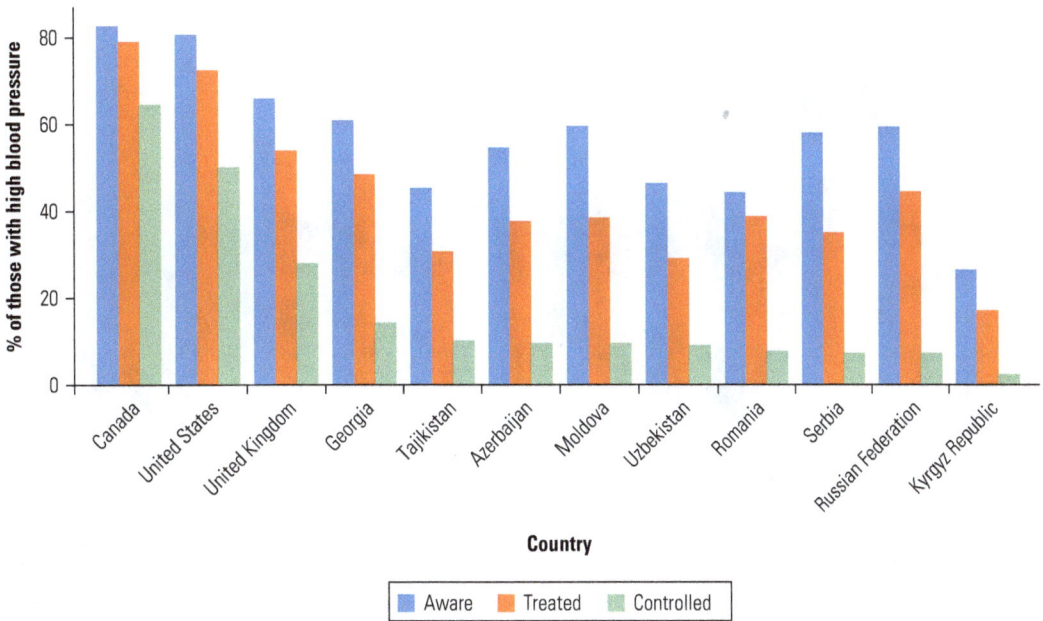

Sources: World Bank 2012a; Egan, Zhao, and Axon 2010; McAlister et al. 2011; Falaschetti et al. 2009; Grujic et al. 2012; Dorobantu et al. 2010; Jakab, Lundeen, and Akkazieva 2007.

There is also evidence of shortcomings in the management of high cholesterol, although here the breakdown appears to take place even earlier in the results chain. That is, many people do not get tested in the first place, a process that requires sending a blood sample to a laboratory for analysis. Figure 3.11 shows that while nearly 40 percent of the adult population in the EU-15 has had a cholesterol test during the previous 12 months, in several ECA countries no more than half that proportion has been tested. As a result, treatment rates are very low. While overtesting for medical conditions can become an important source of inefficiency in health systems, this should be less a concern when the test is relatively cheap and the condition is highly prevalent, as in the case of high cholesterol.

Improving results for hypertension and high cholesterol in principle should not be expensive. It can and should be undertaken mainly in a primary-care setting without high staffing or capital costs. The drugs are also not expensive. Most anti-hypertensives have been off patent for a long time, and the same is increasingly true of statins. The cost effectiveness of drug regimens for

FIGURE 3.11

Cholesterol Testing Can Be Expanded

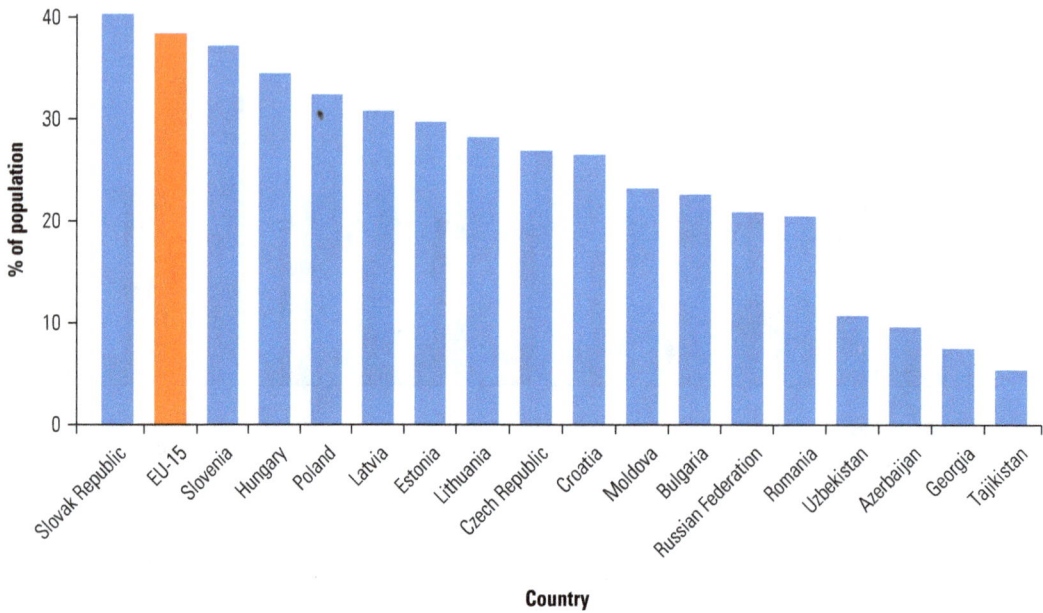

Sources: European Commission 2007; World Bank 2012a.
Note: Figure measures the percentage of respondents who have had a cholesterol test in the past 12 months.

cardiovascular disease has been reviewed favorably as an intervention to promote both health and development more broadly (Gaziano et al. 2006; Jha et al. 2012).

System Measures to Strengthen Primary Care for Heart Disease

Achieving better outcomes through improved control of cardiovascular disease risk factors will require removing barriers to adherence on the patient side and creating stronger incentives on the provider side. There are no guaranteed recipes for improvement, but certain policy initiatives offer promise. Broader institutional reform issues related to primary care are discussed in chapter 6.

On the demand side, an important step toward improving access to drugs and adherence to treatment regimens would be to include basic drugs for cardiovascular disease in outpatient drug benefit packages. Across much of the ECA region, coverage of pharmaceuticals by government or social health insurance plans is lower than in the EU-15, and thus out-of-pocket payments for drugs are high, as discussed in detail in chapter 4. This factor is especially relevant for the CIS region, where the exclusion of outpatient drugs from benefit packages dates back to the pretransition era (Roberts et al. 2010).

The drugs are cheap, and thus the budgetary implications should not be major. While the low costs may be taken as evidence that patients should be able to afford to pay for the drugs themselves, there is growing evidence from the United States that even low copayments for pharmaceutical goods can serve as an effective barrier to access, albeit for "irrational" behavioral reasons. That barrier can even lead to higher downstream systemic costs due to more hospitalization episodes that arise as a result of nonadherence (Baicker and Goldman 2011). This issue is discussed further in box 4.1. Not all drugs may be candidates for expanded coverage, but the case for highly cost-effective drugs for cardiovascular disease appears strong. They hold the promise of huge health gains at the relatively low cost of just a few dollars per patient per month (Lonn et al. 2010).

Lowering financial barriers alone will not solve the adherence problem. People everywhere struggle to follow treatment regimens. But with rates of blood pressure control hovering near 10 percent in most ECA countries, any progress would be welcome. The so-called polypill, a combination drug for treating multiple risk factors, including high blood pressure and cholesterol, could also promote adherence by reducing the complexity of treatment. Making it easier to refill prescriptions can also help.

On the supply side, the challenge is perhaps more complex. Primary-care provision needs to move beyond a generic "heart checkup," as in figure 3.9, to reach closer to the ultimate result of successfully managing risk factors. An increasingly common approach is to implement pay-for-performance (P4P) schemes, whereby medical staff are partially reimbursed on the basis of specific targets or indicators related to outputs instead of inputs. These can provide a significant monetary incentive and, perhaps just as important, a strong signal of what is expected of health workers. In ECA, Armenia and Turkey have very recently launched P4P schemes to help address cardiovascular disease, among other conditions, through primary care. Globally, these schemes have met with varying degrees of success (Maynard 2012; Witter et al. 2012), but the status quo clearly needs to be reassessed.

More generally, managing cardiovascular disease requires important organizational inputs to help patients navigate the health system, especially by ensuring the coordination and continuity of care.

In the absence of these inputs, there may be wide variation in the delivery of care within a country, with little or no link to evidence-based medicine, poor communication between outpatient and inpatient settings, and minimal attention paid to patient self-management. The result will be a higher likelihood of acute episodes, with implications for health outcomes and system costs. To address these shortcomings, strong disease management programs are needed to help establish clear guidelines and patient pathways, institutionalize information flows, and empower patients to take responsibility for their own care. Good examples of such programs adopted recently in Western Europe include those implemented in Germany and the United Kingdom.

At the broader system level, indicators of cardiovascular risk factors could serve as a management tool for benchmarking and monitoring overall health system performance, an area of growing importance for policy makers (Smith et al. 2009). Specific and meaningful "disease content" can be incorporated into broader efforts to strengthen primary care. Managing high blood pressure, the risk factor to which the most deaths in ECA can be attributed, is arguably the most important task of primary care and thus should be a centerpiece of efforts to improve performance.

While the focus has been on cardiovascular disease, many of the key system measures—increasing access to drugs for chronic disease, exploring pay-for-performance to incentivize providers, introducing disease management programs, and using disease-specific indicators to help monitor performance of the health system—apply equally to other conditions. For example, much of this approach also applies to the management of diabetes.

Further into the future, as noted above, progress against heart disease may lead to rising cancer incidence, and cancer-screening rates are still low in much of ECA, including for the most treatable forms (breast, cervical, colon, and prostate). Figure 3.12 shows the details. Substantial progress is now being made against cancer, especially in the United States. Systemic measures for addressing cardiovascular disease will ultimately lend support to the war on cancer.

More broadly, while people in many ECA countries visit the doctor as much as people in the EU-15, those visits do not result in meaningful improvements in chronic disease (especially in primary care), from control of cardiovascular risk factors to cancer screening to other causes. Box 3.4 briefly shifts the focus from mortality to morbidity, where some of the same challenges hold true for the treatment of depression.

FIGURE 3.12

Cancer Screening Is Underprovided in ECA

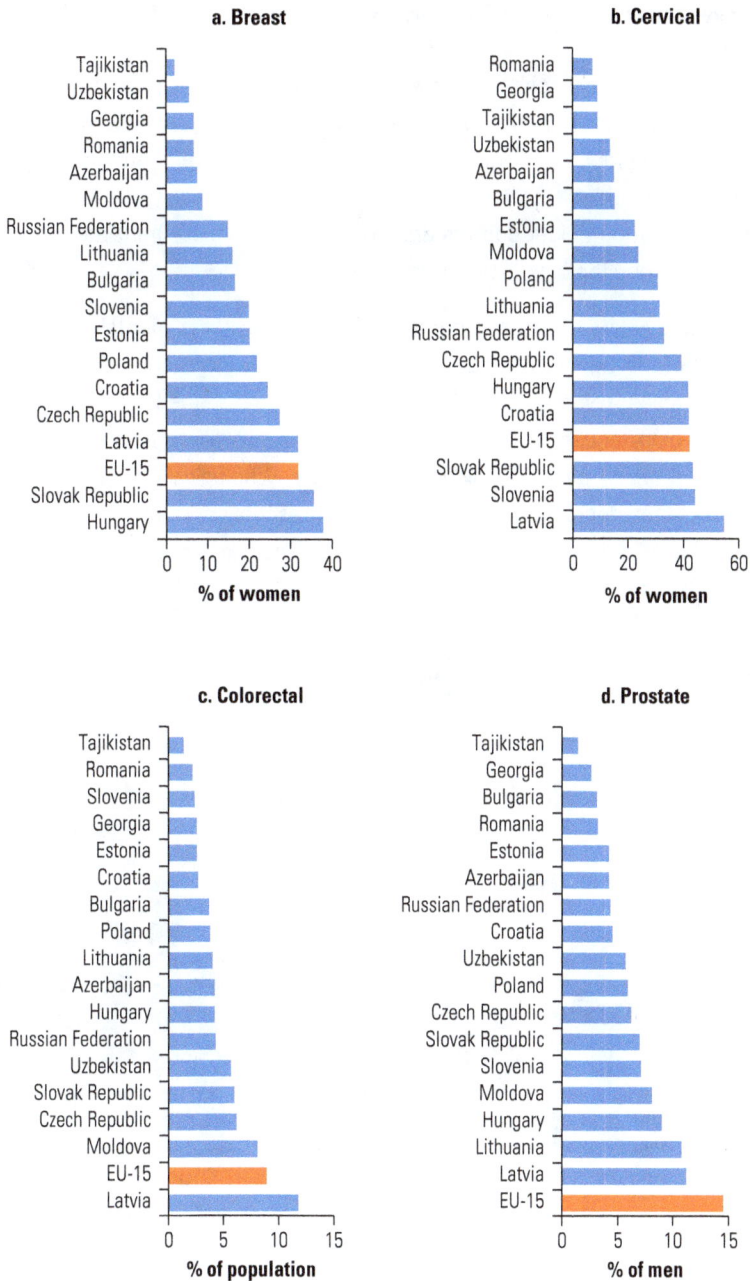

a. Breast

Tajikistan	
Uzbekistan	
Georgia	
Romania	
Azerbaijan	
Moldova	
Russian Federation	
Lithuania	
Bulgaria	
Slovenia	
Estonia	
Poland	
Croatia	
Czech Republic	
Latvia	
EU-15	
Slovak Republic	
Hungary	

% of women

b. Cervical

Romania	
Georgia	
Tajikistan	
Uzbekistan	
Azerbaijan	
Bulgaria	
Estonia	
Moldova	
Poland	
Lithuania	
Russian Federation	
Czech Republic	
Hungary	
Croatia	
EU-15	
Slovak Republic	
Slovenia	
Latvia	

% of women

c. Colorectal

Tajikistan	
Romania	
Slovenia	
Georgia	
Estonia	
Croatia	
Bulgaria	
Poland	
Lithuania	
Azerbaijan	
Hungary	
Russian Federation	
Uzbekistan	
Slovak Republic	
Czech Republic	
Moldova	
EU-15	
Latvia	

% of population

d. Prostate

Tajikistan	
Georgia	
Bulgaria	
Romania	
Estonia	
Azerbaijan	
Russian Federation	
Croatia	
Uzbekistan	
Poland	
Czech Republic	
Slovak Republic	
Slovenia	
Moldova	
Hungary	
Lithuania	
Latvia	
EU-15	

% of men

Sources: European Commission 2007; World Bank 2012a.
Note: Figure shows whether the respondent has been screened for each type of cancer during the past 12 months.
ECA = Europe and Central Asia.

BOX 3.4

Addressing Morbidity Will Require Greater Attention to Mental Health

The focus of this chapter's discussion on health outcomes has been on mortality trends, but there is also a major agenda for addressing morbidity, or sickness and disability. Advances in the treatment of cataracts, arthritis, osteoporosis, and many other conditions have contributed to declining disability rates among the elderly in Western Europe. Replicating those gains in ECA could enhance the quality of life among older cohorts and could also potentially translate into higher labor force participation among those in their 50s and 60s.

However, the largest nonfatal cause of disease burden around the world is mental health (WHO 2008). On this front, there is significant undertreatment in ECA, even though the self-reported prevalence of chronic anxiety or depression is typically higher than in the EU-15 (figure B3.4.1). Populations in the region, especially farther east, are also less likely to consult a primary-care provider or mental health professional "because of a psychological or emotional problem." But they often take anti-depressants, albeit without prescription in many cases. Greater attention to the long-neglected issue of mental health treatment could make a major contribution to improved health outcomes in ECA (Jenkins, Klein, and Parker 2005).

FIGURE B3.4.1
A Higher Burden of Mental Health in ECA

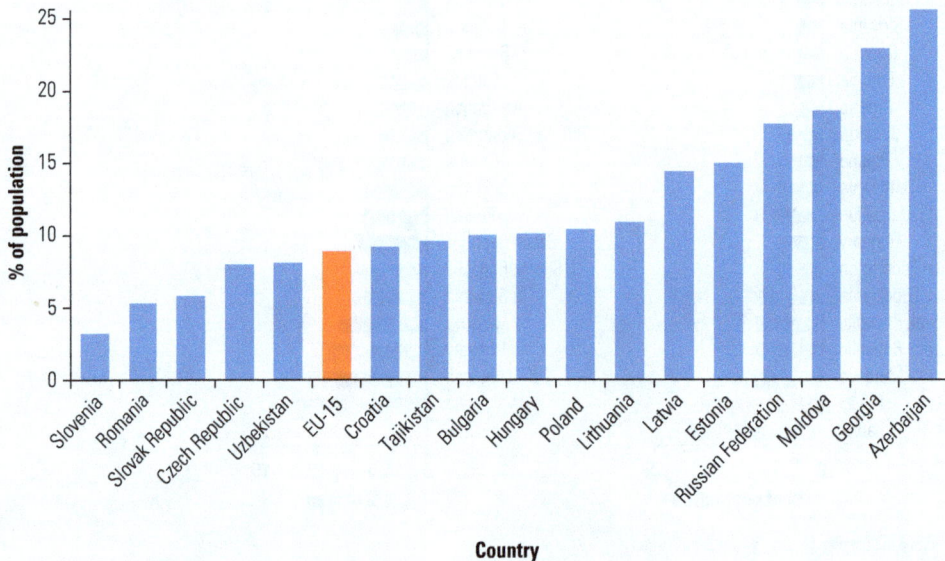

Sources: European Commission 2007; World Bank 2012a.
Note: Figure shows self-reported chronic anxiety or depression, current or previous. ECA = Europe and Central Asia.

The Quality of Treatment and Care for Key Conditions Is Often Poor

Although the main emphasis should be on efforts to prevent illness and manage risk factors, health systems must also aim to achieve a high quality of care in the treatment of chronic and acute episodes of illness. As noted, major health gains have been achieved in advanced health systems in recent decades through better management of heart attack and stroke, from ambulance care and the rapid administration of key drugs to follow-up. The same is true of neonatal care and many other conditions. This section considers health system performance in ECA with regard to quality of care.

There are many definitions of quality of care, including those put forward by Donabedian (1980) and the U.S. Institute of Medicine (2001). While these vary, there is a general consensus that it is multidimensional and comprises three basic elements: structure, clinical process, and outcomes (table 3.1).

For many years, the link between quality of care and population-level health outcomes, while implicit, remained undocumented and unmeasured. However, there is growing evidence on the impact of the quality of care on such outcomes. Evidence shows that the clinical process of care—that is, what health workers actually do when they see their patients—has a stronger association with population health outcomes than structural elements of care. Globally, there is also a growing body of empirical evidence that the quality of care varies significantly, that it is typically inadequate, and that it contributes to the differences in health status across countries and within subgroups of a population (Das, Hammer, and Leonard 2008). It also differs across types of care, providers, and patient characteristics. Thus, understanding the levels, variation, and determinants of the quality of care is important for improving health outcomes.

TABLE 3.1

Three Basic Elements of Quality of Care

Dimension of quality of care	
Structure (inputs)	• Material resources (facilities, drugs, and equipment, for example) • Organization and financing of care (funding, staffing, and payment mechanisms, for example)
Clinical process	• Interactions between health workers and patients in which structural inputs are transformed into health outcomes
Patient outcome	• Clinical outcomes, morbidity, and mortality • Patient satisfaction and responsiveness

Source: Adapted from Peabody et al. 2006.

Hard evidence on the quality of care in ECA countries remains limited, with some exceptions (Peabody et al. 2007; Hill, Chitashvili, and Trevitt 2012). Available information suggests that both the clinical process and the patient outcomes are suboptimal. For example, as indicated in the previous section, hypertension is under control in only about 10 percent of those with high blood pressure in many ECA countries. This common condition is relatively easy to treat with widely available and affordable drugs. Although the causes extend well beyond the clinical setting, one important reason is the low quality of care in the management of this major cardiovascular risk in ECA.

To generate more systematic evidence on the topic for this report, a provider survey was conducted in five countries in the region: Albania, Armenia, Georgia, Russia (Kirov oblast), and Tajikistan. To provide context, it started with the structural aspect of quality by looking at the availability of key inputs for the diagnosis and treatment of common noncommunicable diseases and at maternal and neonatal conditions at the primary and secondary levels and found deficiencies of essential equipment and lab services that are most pronounced for primary care. For example, in Armenia, Georgia, and Tajikistan, primary-care facilities had less than one-third of the essential equipment and basic lab services required for the management of these common conditions.

The main focus of the survey was the clinical process dimension of the quality of care using the approach of clinical performance and value (CPV) vignettes (Peabody et al. 2004). This method attempts to mimic a clinical encounter by presenting health workers with a hypothetical but realistic standardized patient scenario and asks open-ended questions across five domains: patient history, physical exam, ordering tests, diagnosis, and treatment. New information is revealed as the vignette unfolds so that each successive component can be assessed irrespective of previous responses. The objective is to measure provider knowledge as a proxy of the clinical process aspect of quality. The approach has been validated and used in a variety of settings (Peabody et al. 2000). In keeping with this chapter's emphasis on cardiovascular disease and neonatal conditions, the survey used selected tracer conditions to evaluate the competency of health workers in three areas: cardiovascular disease (a patient with multiple risk factors and another with signs of a heart attack), neonatology (birth asphyxia and pneumonia), and obstetrics (postpartum hemorrhage).

The results reveal significant shortcomings in quality of care. The average CPV score was 58 out of a maximum score of 100 (figure 3.13). In most countries, physicians' performance is somewhat lower for cardiovascular disease, especially for a patient with multiple risk factors,

FIGURE 3.13

Quality of Care Can Be Improved for Major Conditions

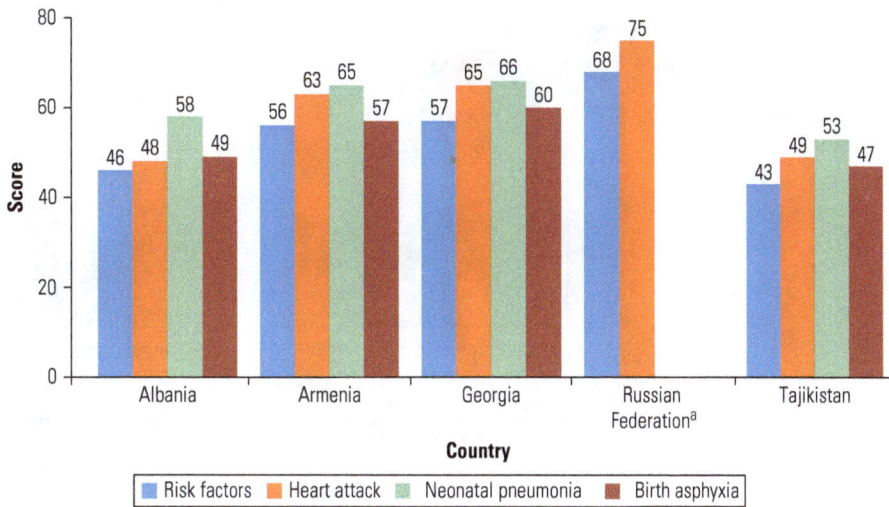

Source: World Bank 2013.
Note: Figure shows average vignette scores of physicians, with a maximum possible score of 100.
a. Results are for Kirov oblast. Neonatal vignettes were not done.

than for neonatal conditions. In the five different domains of a clinical encounter, physician performance was better for history taking (68 percent), conducting physical exams (62 percent), and ordering laboratory tests (62 percent) than for making a diagnosis (49 percent) and giving the right treatment (47 percent). Other key findings that were consistent across countries include: (1) female doctors outperform male doctors; (2) hospitals perform better than primary-care facilities; and (3) specialists score higher than nonspecialists on the CPVs. It is important to note that given the large, well-documented gap between what health providers know and what they do (sometimes referred to as the "know-do gap" in the literature), the actual quality of care in clinical processes for these conditions may be significantly lower than the level indicated by the CPV scores in the survey. In effect, the results represent an upper bound on quality of care.

Underlying these aggregate results is evidence of shortcomings for specific, critical clinical processes. For example, as indicated in figure 3.14, on average across the region 63 percent of doctors surveyed correctly diagnosed a heart attack (70 percent at the hospital level), but with wide cross-country variation in performance. Only 50 and 73 percent, respectively, of hospital workers would give aspirin and sublingual nitrates to a patient with a confirmed diagnosis of heart attack—despite the fact that these cheap and widely available drugs are the universal gold standard in the management of cardiac

FIGURE 3.14

The Quality of Care for Key Health Care Services Can Be Improved

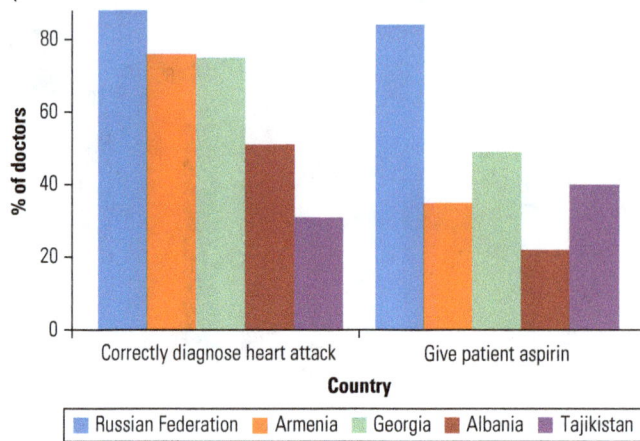

Source: World Bank 2013.
Note: Figure shows provider responses to clinical vignette of heart attack.

emergency. Similar gaps were identified for the treatment of a patient with multiple cardiovascular risk factors. On average, only 65 percent of physicians in the surveyed countries prescribed anti-hypertensive drugs to a hypertensive patient. For high cholesterol, only 49 percent prescribed statins. Albania and Tajikistan especially lag in this respect. Only 19 and 26 percent of Albanian doctors would prescribe cholesterol-lowering and anti-hypertensive drugs, respectively, to patients who need them. This observation is a major cause for concern, given the role that primary care plays in the management of such CVD risks. These findings provide further evidence on the challenge of managing risk factors through primary care as highlighted in the previous section.

Quality of care typically varies widely across facilities and regions within a country, and thus survey findings can highlight the potential gains of raising the standard of care among the lowest performers to that of average or high performers. For example, a vignette-based survey carried out in Ukraine in 2011 revealed very large gaps in quality between the best-performing region, Kiev, and the worst, Crimea. Structural quality measures such as drugs, equipment and supplies, hours of operation, and staffing could not predict this regional variation, but physicians who had recently (within the past year) undergone continuing medical education did have higher scores. Of note, higher-performing physicians were associated with better self-reported health status among patients interviewed at the health clinics.

TABLE 3.2

Summary of Interventions to Improve Quality of Care

Type of interventions	Level of evidence on effectiveness
Interventions changing structural conditions	
Legal mandates, accreditation, and administrative regulations	+
Malpractice litigation to enforce legal mandate	++
Oversight of professional association	++
Clinical guidelines	+++
Targeted education and professional retraining	+++
Organizational change (management models, among others)	++++
Interventions directly affecting provider practices	
Training with peer review feedbacks	+++
Pay-for-performance	++++
High volume of care	++++
Performance-based professional recognition	++++

Source: Adapted from Peabody et al. 2006.
Note: Level of evidence is ranked from "Low" (+) to "High" (++++).

The global body of evidence on effective interventions to improve the quality of care is quite well established (table 3.2), but their application remains limited. For example, a review of the existence of national practice guidelines for selected cardiovascular conditions in three ECA countries in 2011 showed that two did not have any at the national level. In the quality-of-care survey, on average, only 65 percent of hospitals in Armenia, Georgia, Russia (Kirov oblast), and Tajikistan had a committee to oversee quality of care, although such bodies are an essential part of the quality management model. Similarly, about 43 percent of health facilities in these countries had not received any kind of supervisory visit in the past 12 months. Among those that did, only 7 percent of external supervisors had used a checklist to assess the structural quality of care, and only 8 percent had reviewed medical registers. Internal quality control is also deficient, with only about half of all health facilities having applied inventory checklists and medical register audits to themselves, and only half of hospitals had conducted a mortality audit in the event of a death. With regard to continuing medical education, a key intervention commonly used globally to update health workers' professional knowledge and skills, only 38 percent of hospital physicians and 29 percent of primary-care physicians in Tajikistan had received any type of continuing medical training in the past 12 months. For the Kirov oblast in Russia, these rates were 40 and 48 percent, respectively.

In general, there is stronger evidence of an impact on quality when interventions aim to affect provider practices directly and not simply change the structural conditions. An important aspect of this agenda is to better measure provider performance and link it to payment (that is, P4P), professional recognition, and peer review. Experience suggests that nonmonetary incentives can be more powerful than money alone. International benchmarking can also be useful: the OECD already publishes cross-country data on key indicators of quality, such as mortality within 30 days of discharge following a heart attack (OECD 2011). Few ECA countries have national or facility-level data on such indicators.

In summary, there appear to be significant gaps in all three dimensions of quality of care: structure, clinical process, and patient outcomes in the surveyed ECA countries. It is likely that similar challenges exist to varying degrees elsewhere in the region. Improving the quality of care in ECA, especially for the high-burden causes of mortality, such as cardiovascular disease, should be a priority for policy makers.

References

Baicker, K., and D. Goldman. 2011. "Patient Cost-Sharing and Health Care Spending Growth." *Journal of Economic Perspectives* 25 (2): 47–68.

Bhattacharya, J., C. Gathmann, and G. Miller. Forthcoming. "The Gorbachev Anti-Alcohol Campaign and Russia's Mortality Crisis." *American Economic Journal: Applied Economics*.

Black, R. E., S. Cousens, H. L. Johnson, J. E. Lawn, I. Rudan, D. G. Bassani, et al. 2010. "Global, Regional, and National Causes of Child Mortality in 2008: A Systematic Analysis." *Lancet* 375: 1969–87. http://www.thelancet.com/journals/lancet/article/PIIS0140-6736(10)60549-1/fulltext.

Brainerd, E. 2010. "Reassessing the Standard of Living in the Soviet Union: An Analysis Using Archival and Anthropometric Data." *Journal of Economic History* 70 (1): 83–117.

Canudas-Romo, V. 2011. "Mortality Decomposition." Background paper for ECA Regional Health Report, World Bank, Washington, DC.

Cawley, J., and C. Ruhm. 2012. "The Economics of Risky Health Behaviors." In *Handbook of Health Economics*, vol. 2, edited by Mark V. Pauly, Thomas G. McGuire, and Pedro P. Barros, 95–199. Oxford: Elsevier Science BV.

Chaloupka, F., R. Peck, J. Tauras, X. Xu, and A. Yurekli. 2010. "Cigarette Excise Taxation: The Impact of Tax Structure on Prices, Revenues, and Cigarette Smoking." NBER Working Paper 16287, National Bureau of Economic Research, Cambridge, MA.

Countdown. 2012. *Countdown to 2015: Maternal, Newborn, and Child Survival.* Geneva, http://www.countdown2015mnch.org.

Cutler, D. M., A. Rosen, and S. Vijan. 2006. "The Value of Medical Spending in the United States, 1960–2000." *New England Journal of Medicine* 355: 920–27.

Das, J., J. Hammer, and K. Leonard. 2008. "The Quality of Medical Advice in Low-Income Countries." *Journal of Economic Perspectives* 22 (2): 93–114.

Donabedian, A. 1980. *The Definition of Quality and Approaches to Its Assessment.* Ann Arbor, MI: Health Administration Press.

Dorobantu, M., R. O. Darabont, E. Badila, and S. Ghiorghe. 2010. "Prevalence, Awareness, Treatment, and Control of Hypertension in Romania: Results of the SEPHAR Study." *International Journal of Hypertension* (February).

Egan, B., Y. Zhao, and R. N. Axon. 2010. "US Trends in Prevalence, Awareness, Treatment, and Control of Hypertension, 1988–2008." *Journal of the American Medical Association* 303 (20): 2043–50.

EPHA (European Public Health Association). 2012. "European Smoking Bans: Evolution of the Legislation," http://www.epha.org/a/1941.

European Commission. 2007. *Eurobarometer 66.2,* October–November 2006. TNS Opinion & Social, Brussels. GESIS Data Archive ZA4527, dataset version 1.0.

———. 2010. *Eurobarometer 72.3,* October 2009. TNS Opinion & Social, Brussels. GESIS Data Archive ZA4977, dataset version 1.0.

Falaschetti, E., M. Chaudhury, J. Mindell, and N. Poulter. 2009. "Continued Improvement in Hypertension Management in England: Results from the Health Survey for England." *Hypertension* 53: 480–86.

Ford, E. S., U. Ajani, J. Croft, J. Critchley, D. Labarthe, T. Kottke, W. Giles, and S. Capewell. 2007. "Explaining the Decrease in U.S. Deaths from Coronary Disease, 1980–2000." *New England Journal of Medicine* 356: 2388–98.

Garber, A. 2003. "Comparing Health Care Systems from the Disease-Specific Perspective." In *A Disease-Based Comparison of Health Systems.* Paris: OECD.

Gaziano, T., K. S. Reddy, F. Paccaud, S. Horton, and V. Chaturvedi. 2006. "Cardiovascular Disease." In *Disease Control Priorities in Developing Countries,* 2nd ed., edited by D. T. Jamison, J. G. Breman, A. R. Measham, G. Alleyene, M. Claeson, D. B. Evans, et al., 645–62. Oxford: Oxford University Press.

Giovino, G. A., S. Mirza, J. Samet, P. Gupta, M. Jarvis, N. Bhala, R. Peto, W. Zatonski, J. Hsia, J. Morton, K. Palipudi, and S. Asma. 2012. "Tobacco Use in 3 Billion Individuals from 16 Countries: An Analysis of Nationally Representative Cross-Sectional Household Surveys." *Lancet* 380: 668–79.

Gotsadze, G., I. Chikovani, K. Goguadze, D. Balabanova, and M. McKee. 2010. "Reforming Sanitary-Epidemiological Service in Central and Eastern Europe and the Former Soviet Union: An Exploratory Study." *BMC Public Health* 10: 440.

Gruber, J., and B. Koszegi. 2001. "Is Addiction Rational? Theory and Evidence." *Quarterly Journal of Economics* 116 (4): 1261–1303.

Grujic V., N. Dragnic, S. Kvrgic, S. Susnjevic, J. Grujic, and S. Travar. 2012. "Epidemiology of Hypertension in Serbia: Results of a National Survey." *Journal of Epidemiology* 22 (3): 261–66.

Hill, K., T. Chitashvili, and J. Trevitt. 2012. *Assessment of Non-Communicable Disease Prevention, Screening and Care Best Practices for Women of Reproductive Age in Albania, Armenia, Georgia, and Russia.* Washington, DC: University Research Corporation and U.S. Agency for International Development.

Institute of Medicine. 2001. *Crossing the Quality Chasm: A New Health System for the 21st Century.* Washington, DC: National Academy Press.

Jakab, M., E. Lundeen, and B. Akkazieva. 2007. "Health System Effectiveness in Hypertension Control in Kyrgyzstan." Europe Policy Research Paper 44, World Health Organization, Bishkek.

Jenkins, R., J. Klein, and C. Parker. 2005. "Mental Health in Post-Communist Countries." *British Medical Journal* 331 (7510): 173–74.

Jha, P., R. Nugent, S. Verguet, D. Bloom, and R. Hum. 2012. "Copenhagen Consensus 2012 Challenge Paper: Chronic Diseases." http://www.copenhagenconsensus.com/sites/default/files/Chronic%2BDisease.pdf.

Kesternich, I., B. Siflinger, J. P. Smith, and J. K. Winter. 2012. "The Effects of World War II on Economic and Health Outcomes across Europe." RAND Working Paper WR-917, RAND Corporation, Santa Monica, CA.

Kostova, D., H. Ross, E. Blecher, and S. Markowitz. 2010. "Prices and Cigarette Demand: Evidence from Youth Tobacco Use in Developing Countries." NBER Working Paper 15781, National Bureau of Economic Research, Cambridge, MA.

Lawn, J. E., S. Cousens, and J. Zupan. 2005. "4 Million Neonatal Deaths: When? Where? Why?" *Lancet* 365: 891–900.

Laxminarayan, R., A. Mills, J. Breman, A. Measham, G. Alleyne, M. Claeson, P. Jha, P. Musgrove, J. Chow, S. Shahid-Salles, and D. Jamison. 2006. "Advancement of Global Health: Key Messages from the Disease Control Priorities Project." *Lancet* 367 (9517): 1193–1208.

Leon, D., V. Shkolnikov, and M. McKee. 2009. "Alcohol and Russian Mortality: A Continuing Crisis." *Addiction* 104: 1630–36.

Lonn, E., J. Bosch, K. Teo, P. Pais, D. Xavier, and S. Yusuf. 2010. "The Polypill in the Prevention of Cardiovascular Disease." *Circulation* 122: 2078–88.

Mackenbach, J. P., I. Stirbu, A. Roskam, M. Schaap, G. Menvielle, M. Leinsalu, and A. Kunst. 2008. "Socioeconomic Inequalities in Health in 22 European Countries." *New England Journal of Medicine* 358: 2468–81.

Maynard, A. 2012. "The Powers and Pitfalls of Payment for Performance." *Health Economics* 21: 3–12.

McAlister, F., K. Wilkins, M. Joffres, F. Leenen, G. Fodor, M. Gee, M. Tremblay, R. Walker, H. Johansen, and N. Campbell. 2011. "Changes in the Rates of Awareness, Treatment and Control of Hypertension in Canada over the Past Two Decades." *Canadian Medical Association Journal* 183 (9): 1007–13.

Nolte, E., and M. McKee. 2003. "Measuring the Health of Nations: Analysis of Mortality Amenable to Health Care." *British Medical Journal* 327:1129.

———. 2004. *Does Health Care Save Lives? Avoidable Mortality Revisited.* London: Nuffield Trust.

OECD (Organisation for Economic Co-operation and Development). 2010. *Health at a Glance: Europe.* Paris: OECD Publishing.

————. 2011. *Health at a Glance 2011: OECD Indicators.* Paris: OECD Publishing.

Peabody, J., J. Luck, P. Glassman, T. Dresselhouse, and M. Lee. 2000. "Comparison of Vignettes, Standardized Patients, and Chart Abstraction: A Prospective Validation Study of Three Methods for Measuring Quality." *Journal of the American Medical Association* 283 (13): 1715–22.

Peabody, J., J. Luck, P. Glassman, S. Jain, J. Jansen, M. Spell, et al. 2004. "Measuring the Quality of Physician Practice by Using Clinical Vignettes: A Prospective Validation Study." *Annals of Internal Medicine* 141 (10): 771–80.

Peabody, J., R. J. Nordyke, F. Tozija, J. Luck, J. A. Munoz, and A. Sunderland, et al. 2007. "Quality of Care and Its Impact on Population Health: A Cross-Sectional Study in Macedonia." *Social Science and Medicine* 62: 2216–24.

Peabody, J., M. M. Taguiwalo, D. A. Robalino, and J. Frenk. 2006. "Improving the Quality of Care in Developing Countries." In *Disease Control Priorities in Developing Countries,* edited by D. Jamison, J. G. Breman, A. R. Measham, G. Alleyene, M. Claeson, and D. B. Evans, 1293–1308. Oxford: Oxford University Press.

Rechel, B., L. Shapo, and M. McKee. 2005. "Are the Health Millennium Development Goals Appropriate for Eastern Europe and Central Asia?" *Health Policy* 73: 339–51.

Roberts, B., A. Gilmore, A. Stickley, D. Rotman, V. Prohoda, C. Haerpfer, and M. McKee. 2012. "Changes in Smoking Prevalence in Eight Countries of the Former Soviet Union between 2001 and 2010." *American Journal of Public Health* 102 (7): 1320–28.

Roberts B., A. Stickley, D. Balabanova, and M. McKee. 2010. "Irregular Treatment of Hypertension in the Former Soviet Union." *Journal of Epidemiology and Community Health.* http://jech.bmj.com/content/early/2010/11/04/jech.2010.111377.abstract.

Sloan, F. A., J. Ostermann, C. Conover, D. H. Taylor, Jr., and G. Picone. 2004. *The Price of Smoking.* Cambridge, MA: MIT Press.

Smith, P., E. Mossialos, I. Papanicolas, and S. Leatherman, eds. 2009. *Performance Measurement for Health System Improvement: Experiences, Challenges, and Prospects.* Cambridge: Cambridge University Press.

Spinney, L. 2007. "Public Smoking Bans Show Signs of Success in Europe." *Lancet* 369 (9572): 1507–508.

Stickley, A., Y. Razvodovsky, and M. McKee. 2009. "Alcohol Mortality in Russia: A Historical Perspective." *Public Health* 123: 20–26.

Treisman, D. 2010. "Death and Prices: The Political Economy of Russia's Alcohol Crisis." *Economics of Transition* 18 (2): 281–331.

Tunstall-Pedoe, H., D. Vanuzzo, M. Hobbs, M. Mähönen, Z. Cepatis, K. Kuulasmaa, and U. Keil. 2000. "Estimation of Contribution of Changes in Coronary Care to Improving Survival, Event Rates, and Coronary Heart Disease Mortality across the WHO MONICA Project Populations." *Lancet* 355: 688–700.

UNAIDS (United Nations Programme on HIV/AIDS). 2012. *Together We Will End AIDS.* Geneva: United Nations Programme on HIV/AIDS.

UNECE (United Nations Economic Conference for Europe). 2012. *The UN Economics Commission for Europe Report on Achieving the Millennium Development Goals in Europe and Central Asia.* Geneva: United Nations Economic Conference for Europe.

UNGASS (United Nations General Assembly Special Session). 2010. *Country Progress Reports for the Russian Federation and Ukraine.* Geneva: United Nations General Assembly Special Session.

UNICEF (United Nations Children's Fund). 2010. Childinfo (database), United Nations Children's Fund, New York, http://www.childinfo.org.

Vallin, J., and F. Mesle. 2001. *Trends in Mortality and Differential Mortality.* Population Studies 36. Strasbourg: Council of Europe Publishing.

Wang, H., J. Sindelar, and S. Busch. 2006. "The Impact of Tobacco Expenditure on Household Consumption Patterns in Rural China." *Social Science and Medicine* 62: 1414–26.

WHO (World Health Organization). 2004. *World Report on Road Traffic Injury Prevention.* Geneva: WHO.

———. 2008. *Global Burden of Disease: 2004 Update.* Geneva: World Health Organization.

———. 2009a. *Global Status Report on Road Safety.* Geneva: World Health Organization.

———. 2009b. *Global Health Risks: Mortality and Burden of Disease Attributable to Selected Major Risks.* Geneva: World Health Organization.

———. 2010. World Health Statistics (database), Geneva, World Health Organization, http://www.who.int/topics/statistics/en/.

———. 2011a. *WHO Report on the Global Tobacco Epidemic.* Geneva: World Health Organization.

———. 2011b. *Global Status Report on Alcohol and Health.* Geneva: World Health Organization.

———. 2012a. *Alcohol in the European Union: Consumption, Harm, and Policy Approaches.* Geneva: World Health Organization.

———. 2012b. Health for All (database), Geneva, World Health Organization, http://www.euro.who.int/en/what-we-do/data-and-evidence/databases/european-health-for-all-database-hfa-db2.

Witter, S., A. Fretheim, F. Kessy, and A. Lindahl. 2012. "Paying for Performance to Improve the Delivery of Health Interventions in Low- and Middle-Income Countries." *Cochrane Database of Systematic Reviews*, Issue 2. http://onlinelibrary.wiley.com/doi/10.1002/14651858.CD007899.pub2/otherversions.

World Bank. 2005. *Dying Too Young: Addressing Premature Mortality and Ill Health due to Non-Communicable Diseases and Injuries in the Russian Federation.* Washington, DC: World Bank.

———. 2012a. "Findings from a Household Survey on Health in Six ECA Countries." Draft. World Bank, Washington, DC.

———. 2012b. "Health Equity and Financial Protection Data-sheets for ECA." World Bank, Washington, DC.

———. 2013. "The Quality of Care in ECA: Findings from a Five-Country Study." World Bank, Washington, DC.

CHAPTER 4

Improving Financial Protection and Equity: A Safety Net for All

Key Messages

- High out-of-pocket payments are a concern if they impose significant consumption risk on households, if they result in high inequality in access to care, or if they reflect rent seeking by providers at the expense of the population using health care.

- To help overcome behavioral biases toward underuse of preventive care, a lower degree of patient cost sharing may be more desirable for key preventive services (including some pharmaceuticals) than traditional approaches allow.

- Once the various reasons to achieve lower OOP spending are summed up, theory and evidence suggest that less than 25 percent of total health financing drawn from this source is a reasonable policy objective. OOP spending in many ECA countries is between 40 and 70 percent, while the EU-15 average is 18 percent.

- Households in ECA's high OOP-payment countries are spending significantly more on health, and with a higher variance, than counterparts in EU-15 countries; a large share of this OOP spending is on drugs.

- The incidence of catastrophic health expenditures and inequality of utilization is higher in countries that rely heavily on OOP spending for health financing; over half of all OOP spending is catastrophic in most countries.

- How much a government spends on health matters a lot for the degree of financial protection achieved by a health system, but higher spending does not automatically translate into improved financial protection outcomes.

- Rent seeking by providers in the form of informal payments and high pharmaceutical price markups are important causes of weak financial protection in ECA.

- To improve financial protection, the policy agenda will require some combination of increased health budgets and supply-side measures to address informal payments and high drug spending.

- Special effort should be made to ensure that improvements in financial protection benefit the poorest first, for example, through targeted health programs.

The previous chapter explored the policy agenda for improving on recent trends with respect to health outcomes in Europe and Central Asia (ECA). In this chapter, we shift our attention to the equally challenging issue of how to pay for it. People want better health, but they want many other things too, and more money spent on health means less is available for everything else. We begin with the household perspective—avoiding undue financial distress on individuals in the course of obtaining health care—and in the next chapter, we focus on the same topic from the perspective of maintaining a sustainable government health budget.

The major focus of attention with respect to financial protection is out-of-pocket (OOP) payments for health by households at the point of care. How much is being spent, for what, by whom, and to whom? And what are the causes, consequences, and policy implications of these payments? This chapter aims to address these questions.

As shown in chapter 1, the long-term trend in out-of-pocket payments for health financing in ECA is a mixed picture, with some countries making good progress in reducing OOP payments to more moderate levels, while many others are not. About half the countries in the region have either increased their reliance on OOP payments significantly since 1997 (the earliest year for which reliable cross-country data are available) or maintain persistently high levels. In brief, taking the region as a whole, there has been very little convergence with the EU-15 on this key performance indicator. This chapter focuses on how a more rapid convergence in that regard might be achieved to mitigate the impact of high OOP payments on households.

The chapter begins with a brief overview of conceptual issues related to OOP payments. It then examines some empirical evidence on OOP spending drawn from household surveys, with a focus on five key stylized facts. The final section offers a diagnosis of some of the main causes of weak financial protection in those countries that continue to struggle with this issue and discusses some policy options that can help improve financial protection in the region. It also looks at some case studies of success.

The Problem with Out-of-Pocket Payments: Conceptual Issues

Out-of-pocket spending for health care by households takes place when a health expense is either not (fully) subsidized or not (fully) reimbursed through government funding or through insurance. Such spending can include full payment by the patient if a service is not included in a formal benefit package (if indeed such a thing exists), as well as partial contributions in the form of copayments, deductibles, or coinsurance. The payments may be "formal"—that is, part of an official policy of cost sharing—or "informal" if the payment does not adhere to some official rule. In practice, the distinction between formal and informal payments is often not very clear.

Health Spending Is Different: Confronting Consumption Risk, Externalities, Equity, and Rent-Seeking

For most goods and services, household spending patterns are presumed to be a matter of individual choice, and there is little reason to believe that these outcomes can be improved on or should otherwise be the focus of policy intervention. But health expenditures are different from most other household purchases for several reasons.

First, the uncertainty and potentially high cost associated with health expenditures—we do not know when we might fall sick or how much it will cost if we do—make them amenable to prepayment and risk-pooling arrangements. There are few if any other significant items in a typical household budget that are subject to such uncertainty in demand. Lifetime health costs also vary widely. By making small regular contributions to future health care needs through taxes or insurance premiums, a household will be better off than if it were to face the risk of large, unpredictable out-of-pocket health payments when a household member falls sick. In economic jargon, an inability to smooth consumption directly reduces welfare and may lead to informal risk-management strategies (for example, borrowing or selling assets) that can hinder productive activity. Even if consumption is smoothed in the face of a health shock, the manner of doing so may impose its own burden. Thus, one of the most important sources of economic risk faced by households is unexpected illness (Townsend 1995; Gertler and Gruber 2002; Chetty and Looney 2006).

Second, in the case of preventing and treating infectious disease, there is a potential benefit not just for the individual, but for society as a whole. Thus, subsidized health care makes sense in addressing the externalities. In ECA, HIV/AIDS and tuberculosis are important examples.

Third, access to health care is often viewed as something that should not be determined primarily by ability to pay or by wealth. Most societies are less willing to accept large inequalities in health care than, for example, in the ownership of common consumer goods, a view reflected in some of the survey evidence in chapter 2. Lowering financial barriers in the form of OOP payments can help reduce health inequalities. This rationale underlies the notion of "social" health insurance, with contributions based on income or wages so that better-off households contribute more, while health care utilization is in principle based on need.

Fourth, health care goods and services are often complex products, and the assumption of a well-informed consumer making a rational choice to buy services in a competitive market according to individual preference is difficult to maintain (Arrow 1963). Patients typically do not have the knowledge or expertise to diagnose and treat their illness or to judge the quality of care received. Moreover, in a state of illness they are usually not in a position to shop around for better quality or lower prices. When the life of a family member is in peril, people may be persuaded to pay for care "no matter the cost." Hospitals, laboratories, and drug companies may also have significant market power. As a result, providers can take advantage of their superior knowledge and advantageous position to charge for unnecessary additional services, higher prices, or both. In short, high OOP payments may reflect rent seeking by providers.

However, while these issues highlight conditions under which out-of-pocket payments may be undesirable, the complete elimination of such payments is unlikely to be good policy either. Some services may not warrant any subsidization (cosmetic surgery, for example), while others may be too expensive to cover the entire population in lower-income countries (some cancer treatments, for example), but in both cases those who are willing and able to pay out of pocket should not be prevented from doing so. OOP payments can also be an important tool for creating greater patient responsibility for the costs of health care, for better aligning the benefits and costs of each health care dollar spent, and thus for achieving a more sustainable health-spending trajectory. The challenge is to design a benefit package that achieves a balance among numerous considerations, including the rationale for public spending, clinical evidence, available fiscal resources, and efficiency and equity concerns.

The issue of optimal cost sharing is a complex one, and a growing body of evidence suggests that *less* patient cost sharing may be desirable for a broader range of services than traditionally believed. This problem is discussed further in box 4.1. Once the various reasons for achieving lower OOP payments are summed up, theory and evidence suggest that less than 25 percent of total health financing drawn from this source is a reasonable policy objective. In the EU-15, for example, the ratio is 18 percent.

When Is Financial Protection a Problem?

A graphic illustration can help convey some of the concepts described here and introduce some common metrics of financial protection (O'Donnell et al. 2008). Figure 4.1 shows a distribution of households in two countries, ranked along the horizontal axis by total monthly consumption from poorest to richest. The vertical drip lines represent OOP spending on health. The poverty line is also shown. The frequency with which households face high health costs—as indicated when they account for a large share of total household expenses—is clearly greater in the panel on the right, suggesting a health system characterized by comparatively weaker financial protection. The figure helps illustrate the two measures commonly used to assess the level of financial protection, namely, the incidence of so-called catastrophic and impoverishing health expenditures.

Optimal Cost-Sharing for Health: How Much Should Patients Pay Out of Pocket?

How do we balance the problems of too much health-spending risk (due to too little coverage) with too much health care use (due to overly generous coverage)? The trade-off between risk protection and moral hazard is one of the classic issues addressed in health economics (Pauly 1968; Zeckhauser 1970). A risk-averse individual would prefer the certainty of paying a fixed insurance premium to facilitate consumption smoothing rather than face the risk of a very high out-of-pocket payment in the event of a health shock. By so doing, he or she can effectively transfer income from a "good" health state to a "bad" health state. However, reducing the cost of health care at the point of service to zero or close to it may invite overuse (that is, marginal benefits lower than marginal cost). As a result, having no insurance would expose households to excessive risk, while full insurance would lead to overconsumption of health care. "Optimal health insurance," including some OOP spending through cost sharing, would balance these two factors. Standard theory suggests that lower-cost, more certain spending items such as some pharmaceuticals should be subject to higher cost sharing, because the value of insurance in these cases is lower. Also, copayments should be higher for services with higher demand elasticity, because the resulting cost of overconsumption is higher.

But a growing body of evidence is casting doubt on this standard approach and lends support to the view that optimal cost sharing in many important cases should often be lower than commonly argued. First, there are many different health care goods, and cost-sharing policies applied to one will affect the consumption of others. For example, higher OOP payment for physician visits and anti-hypertensive drugs may lead to lower patient adherence and thus to more frequent unnecessary hospitalizations for hypertension, with consequent costs to the system. In other words, it is not only own-price elasticities that matter but also cross-price elasticities. Empirical work in the United States has uncovered many examples of this phenomenon at work (Baicker and Goldman 2011). It appears to be particularly relevant in the case of pharmaceuticals and has an impact on aggregate spending. These findings have important policy implications for ECA, where drugs commonly represent the largest share of total OOP spending.

Second, while the moral hazard argument emphasizes overuse, the psychology and behavioral economics literature highlights the problem of underuse, with far-reaching consequences for the received wisdom on optimal health insurance (Baicker, Mullainathan, and Schwartzstein 2012). Heart patients may forgo their cholesterol-lowering drug, or diabetics may skip an insulin dose, because they "feel OK right now"; someone else may postpone a doctor visit because he or she can always "go tomorrow" but may never do so; yet another might disregard a cancer-screening program because the process is unpleasant or may bring bad news. These are not insignificant examples: they are representative of the very chronic diseases that account for the vast majority of ECA's disease burden.

continued

BOX 4.1 *continued*

In brief, people do not always make rational choices. Our decision-making capacities may be particularly challenged when facing uncertainty, balancing short-term costs with long-term benefits, and processing complexity—all of which are common in the health care arena. Lowering the OOP cost of care in the examples above will not automatically solve the problem, but it would help eliminate one possible barrier. In fact, in some cases negative prices (incentive payments, for example) may be justified. Nonprice interventions, such as reminding patients with chronic diseases by phone about doctor visits, can also help. Public spending to mitigate the private costs incurred by individuals as a result of their own suboptimal choices might raise some objections from those who prefer a minimalist approach. But the fact that these choices can also affect systemwide costs (that is, monetary externalities) is also important.

What does this mean for policies related to OOP spending? First, it suggests that traditional views of optimal cost sharing need to be reconsidered, as greater subsidization of certain important types of care may be warranted. Second, combining the standard argument to reduce catastrophic risk with the newer behavioral concepts discussed here helps bring theory closer in line with the observed reality in most advanced countries: that is, OOP payments accounting for less than a quarter of total health spending (Liebman and Zeckhauser 2008). Third, there are still ways to seek better balance. For example, the concept of "value-based cost sharing" suggests applying lower or no copayments for services known to be of high value, such as preventive care visits or basic pharmaceuticals, and higher copayments for services with lower therapeutic value (Chernew, Rosen, and Fendrick 2007). A policy of means-tested exemptions, possibly with broader population coverage, also remains relevant.

FIGURE 4.1
What Does Financial Protection Look Like?

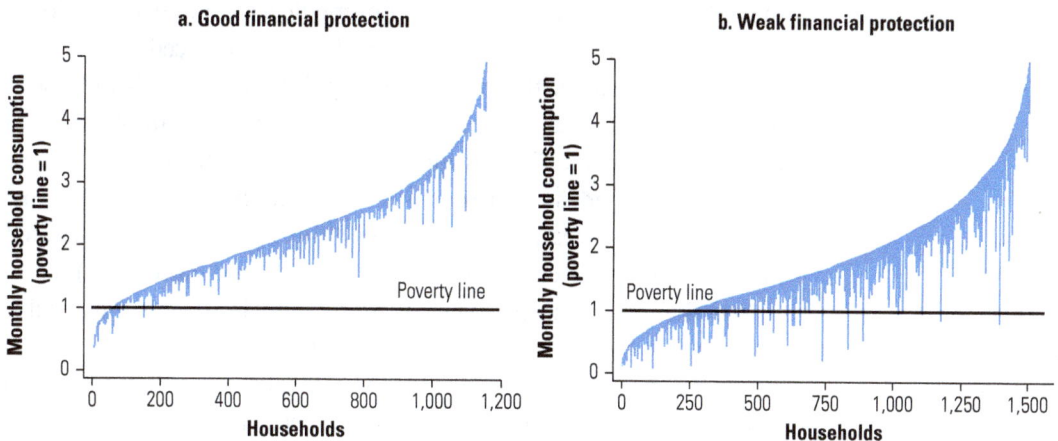

Source: World Bank staff.
Note: Households are ordered from poorest to richest; vertical lines represent out-of-pocket health payments.

The occurrence of high OOP spending is commonly referred to as "catastrophic" health expenditures when they exceed some threshold share of either total or nonfood expenditure. Using survey data to estimate the incidence of catastrophic health expenditures is a common method for measuring financial protection and making cross-country comparisons. The choice of threshold is somewhat arbitrary, but a common practice is to examine a range of thresholds, typically 10–25 percent of total consumption expenditure or 25–40 percent of nonfood expenditure. Catastrophic episodes can often account for well over half of health spending. Some empirical evidence is presented in the next section.

High out-of-pocket payments for health may also cause a household to fall below the poverty line—that is, they can be "impoverishing." If a household has total consumption expenditures (pre-OOP) above the national poverty line but its total nonmedical spending (post-OOP) is below the poverty line, it could be considered to have suffered impoverishment due to OOP spending for health. As in the case of catastrophic OOP spending, impoverishment is evidently a more frequent occurrence in the country depicted in the right-hand panel of figure 4.1. Unlike the catastrophic measure, the concept of impoverishing OOP spending puts the emphasis on crossing the poverty line irrespective of the size of payments. This method is another common way to measure the degree of financial protection provided by a country's health system.

A common underlying assumption of these concepts is that health spending is generally nondiscretionary, an interpretation that is supported by evidence that the income elasticity for health is typically quite low (Deaton and Zaidi 2002). Hence, the rationale for measuring impoverishment due to OOP spending is that a household below the poverty line on the basis of its nonmedical spending alone would not have been poor if the illness episode had not forced it to pay for health care. Instead, the household could have used this money to buy items that actually add to its well-being, rather than restore it to its pre-illness level. This distinction between nonhealth and health spending—one adds to current welfare while the other replaces lost welfare—is why health-related expenditures are often not included in consumption-based estimates of poverty (World Bank 2005).

Whether the concepts of catastrophic and impoverishing health spending are an accurate way to evaluate the true impact of OOP payments is a matter for debate, since in reality, households are likely to resort to several possible coping mechanisms that would allow for consumption smoothing, such as drawing down savings, borrowing, or selling assets. Thus, a costly illness episode in one period would not necessarily have an immediate and commensurate impact on total consumption in the same period. But it is difficult to say since we do not observe counterfactual spending. A more dynamic assessment of household impact can be undertaken with data capturing household consumption patterns before, during, and after a health shock. Some methods have been proposed to adjust the "raw" catastrophic estimates accordingly, and these suggest a smaller impact of OOP spending on households (Flores et al. 2008). But borrowed money has to be paid back eventually, distressed asset sales result in forgone revenue streams, and if health shocks are correlated over time—as would be expected for those with chronic diseases—then the financial burden will only accumulate (Wagstaff 2008). A key benefit of insurance mechanisms for low-income households in developing countries is not consumption smoothing itself but rather reducing the use of inefficient smoothing methods (Chetty and Looney 2007).

While measures of financial protection are not perfect, we will use the concepts presented here as the basis for the empirical work in the next section. They do not fully capture the coping mechanisms or the care forgone by individuals who never sought health care precisely because OOP spending is too high. Nor do they capture the lost earnings that may result from the health shock. Despite their flaws, such measures are useful for international comparisons of the degree of financial protection afforded by various health systems.

A Greater Reliance on Out-of-Pocket Payments Results in More Catastrophic Payments and Higher Inequality

To generate empirical evidence on the conceptual issues discussed in the previous section, a detailed analysis of recent household surveys in 11 ECA countries was undertaken (Ali and Smith 2012). These countries include most of those identified in chapter 1 with either a persistently high level of OOP payments since the 1990s or a significant increase in reliance on OOP spending over the same period. In this section, we present and discuss five key stylized facts emerging from this analysis. The results update and add to a large existing literature on financial protection in ECA (Falkingham, Akkazieva, and Baschieri 2010; Bredenkamp, Mendola, and Gragnolati 2011; Belli, Gotsadze, and Shahriari 2004; Waters et al. 2008; Tomini and Packard 2011; Habicht et al. 2006). Where possible, the results are compared with EU-15 countries (van Doorslaer and Masseria 2004; van Doorslaer, Koolman, and Jones 2004; Lambrelli and O'Donnell 2009; OECD 2011).

The empirical results capture a snapshot of household-level financial protection indicators in recent years. Ideally, we could analyze national trends over time based on similar or identical survey instruments and assess them in the context of policy developments, but for most countries, these data do not exist. Instead, we rely on the most recent snapshots available, in tandem with aggregate indicators on the evolution of reliance on OOP spending over time presented earlier, to highlight the policy agenda.

The first stylized fact is that the average share of total household budgets spent on health varies widely across countries. In Western Europe, this ratio is about 3 percent on average, and a similar level is observed in many new EU member states. However, this share is over 5 percent in eight of the ECA countries analyzed, and in Azerbaijan, Georgia, and Ukraine, it is about 10 percent or higher (figure 4.2). Perhaps more important than the averages is the greater variance in the share of OOP spending among households within these countries—an indication that such spending is a significant source of uncertainty and risk for households.

The second stylized fact is that a large share of total OOP spending is accounted for by drugs (figure 4.3). Across 11 countries, this proportion ranges from 34 percent in Armenia to about 75 percent in Bulgaria and Moldova. The comparable figure for the EU-15 is about

FIGURE 4.2

Many Households in ECA Spend a Greater Share of Their Budgets on Health than Do Households in the EU-15

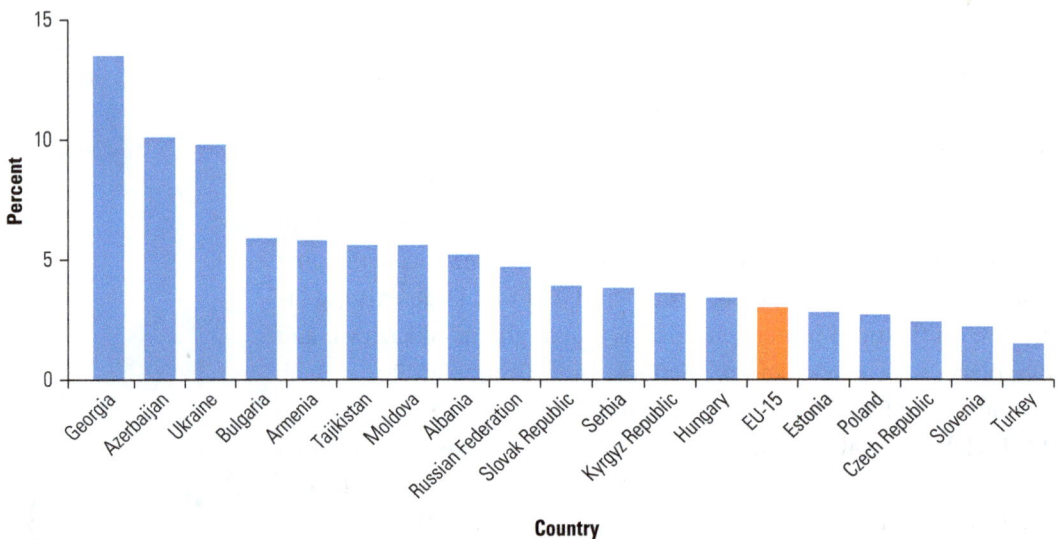

Source: Ali and Smith 2012.
Note: Figure shows out-of-pocket payments on health care as a percentage of total household spending.

FIGURE 4.3

Drugs Account for a Major Share of OOP Spending in Most Countries in ECA

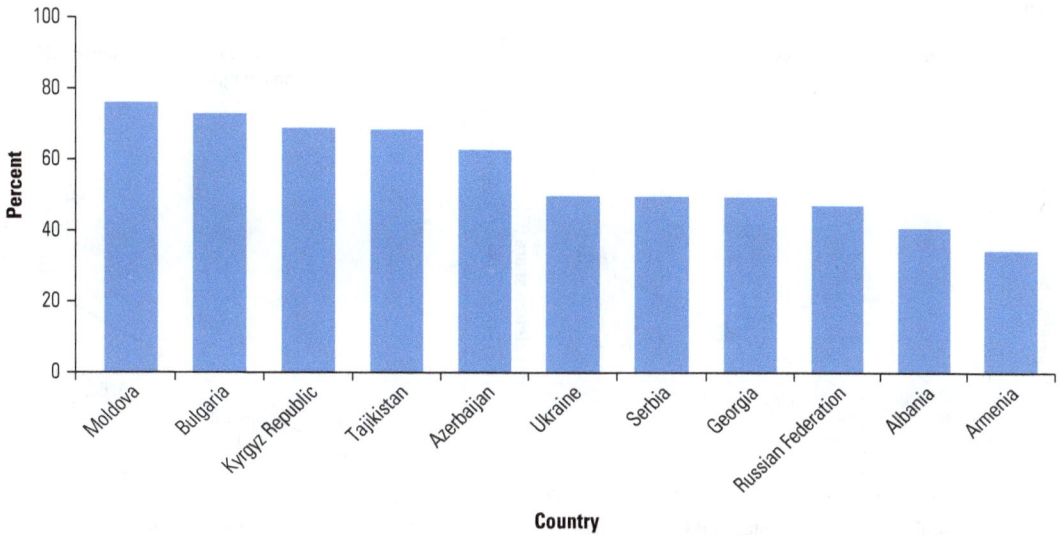

Source: Ali and Smith 2012.
Note: Figure shows out-of-pocket payments on drugs as a percentage of total OOP spending. OOP = out-of-pocket; ECA = Europe and Central Asia.

28 percent, reflecting better coverage of drugs in their benefit packages (see also chapter 6). Within the Organisation for Economic Co-operation and Development (OECD), the highest share of out-of-pocket drug spending by a wide margin is in Estonia and Poland. In ECA, the coexistence of large OOP shares allocated to drugs and frequent occurrences of catastrophic OOP spending (as described below) suggests that the costs of managing chronic disease treatments impose a large financial burden on many households in the region. But there may also be overconsumption of pharmaceuticals in many countries. The challenge of high drug OOP spending is discussed in greater detail below.

The third stylized fact is that a large share of households in ECA faces catastrophic OOP expenditures. As noted, these occur when a household's health spending exceeds some threshold of either total or nonfood expenditure. In the EU-15, the headcount of those who live in households spending more than 10 percent of total expenditures on health is 5.8 percent of the population. In all ECA countries studied, that ratio is above 10 percent, and in five countries higher than 20 percent. This percentage is also notably higher than in East Asia, where the average across 12 countries was about 8 percent, although they generally have younger populations than ECA (van Doorslaer et al. 2007). An alternative threshold of households spending over 25 percent of consumption on health yields a similar pattern, and the same applies if we look at shares of nonfood consumption.

FIGURE 4.4

A Greater Reliance on OOP Payments Is Associated with Higher Incidence of Catastrophic Spending

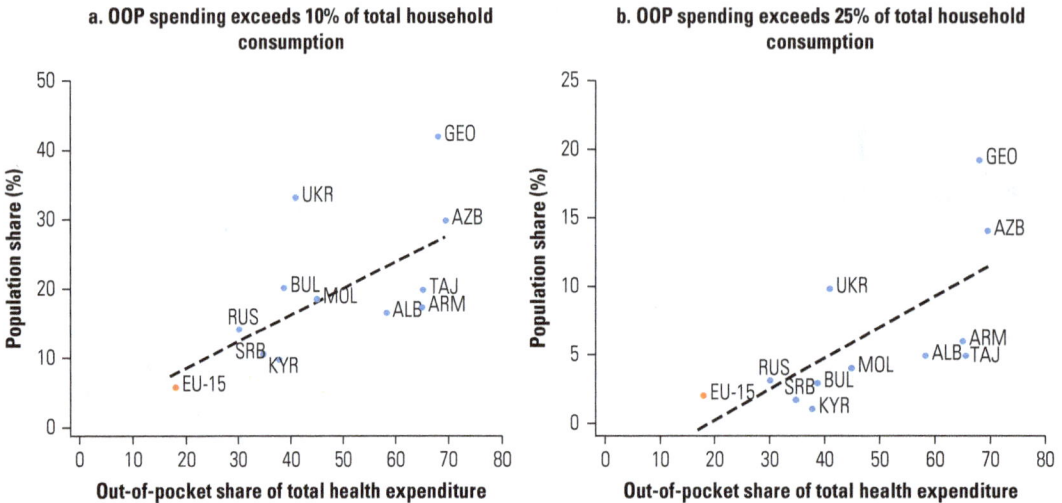

a. OOP spending exceeds 10% of total household consumption

b. OOP spending exceeds 25% of total household consumption

Source: Ali and Smith 2012.
Note: OOP = out-of-pocket.

As shown in figure 4.4, the incidence of catastrophic spending is correlated with a country's overall reliance on OOP payments for health financing. Approximately half the cross-country variation in the incidence of catastrophic spending above 10 percent can be explained by the OOP share of total health expenditures. Previous work shows that the same associations are also observed in Asia and globally (van Doorslaer et al. 2006, 2007; Xu et al. 2010). Once reliance on OOP spending exceeds 30 percent of total health expenditure, there is a marked increase in the incidence of catastrophic spending in health systems around the world.

Moreover, a large share of the monetary value of total OOP spending in a country is catastrophic. For example, between 50 and 80 percent of total OOP spending was incurred by households for which it exceeded 10 percent of their total expenditures. The share of total OOP payments that was catastrophic is somewhat lower in countries with less total OOP spending (for example, Bulgaria, the Russian Federation, and Serbia) and higher in those with more total OOP spending (such as Azerbaijan, Georgia, and Ukraine). Thus, a country that resolves to address "only" catastrophic OOP spending would need to tackle the major share of total OOP payments. This finding is consistent with some of the best available evidence on health care demand from the U.S.-based RAND health insurance experiment, according to which a "catastrophic-only" insurance package results in total expenditures that are nearly 70 percent of those incurred under an "everything covered" package (Manning et al. 1987).

In addition to a high incidence of catastrophic OOP payments, some countries also have many cases of impoverishing OOP spending. Based on an international poverty line of US$2.50 per day, the poverty headcount is between 1.5 and 3 percentage points higher in Armenia, Azerbaijan, the Kyrgyz Republic, Moldova, Tajikistan, and Ukraine as a result of out-of-pocket payments for health. In Georgia, poverty is over 5 percentage points higher. In Bulgaria, Russia, and Serbia, it is below 1 percentage point, reflecting stronger financial protection and higher incomes.

As noted, longitudinal data would allow for a more complete picture of how households are affected by high OOP payments for health. In its absence, some qualitative data can help shed light on this question. For example, about 18 percent of survey respondents in the Kyrgyz Republic reported that they borrowed, sold livestock, drew down savings, or reduced consumption to help finance large health payments during the previous year. A recently available database indicates that several ECA countries that rely heavily on OOP spending also have a much higher than average share of households reporting an outstanding loan for health reasons (Demirguc-Kunt and Klapper 2012).

The fourth stylized fact is that catastrophic spending is more frequent among better-off households in ECA, but not enormously so. The national averages shown in figure 4.4 mask this variation across socioeconomic groups. Concentration indexes of catastrophic spending episodes at the 10 percent threshold are slightly positive in most countries, meaning that these are somewhat more common among richer households. They are most common among the rich, by a wide margin, in Armenia. But they are negative—indicating more catastrophic spending among the poor—in Bulgaria and Russia.

The final stylized fact is that a higher reliance on OOP spending is associated with greater inequality in the use of health care services for both outpatient and inpatient care, as shown in figure 4.5. Again, this factor is measured using a concentration index. Whereas utilization is quite equal across socioeconomic groups in the EU-15 (and in the case of inpatient care, somewhat pro-poor), it is far more unequal in the high OOP spending countries of Albania, Moldova, and Ukraine and in the three countries of the south Caucasus. Inequality in utilization across both outpatient and inpatient settings also suggests that the benefit incidence of public spending is pro-rich.

These results do not adjust for actual need, and since the poor are usually in worse health than the better-off, they tend to understate

FIGURE 4.5

A Greater Reliance on OOP Spending Results in Higher Inequalities in Utilization

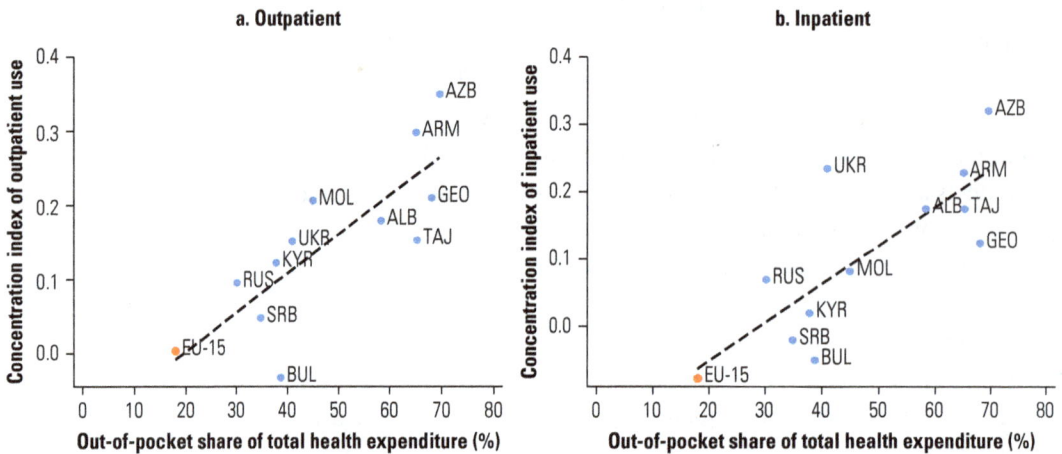

a. Outpatient

b. Inpatient

Source: Ali and Smith 2012.
Note: OOP = out of pocket.

the prevailing degree of inequality in health use. It is important to note that the presence of inequality in the *quality* of care provided to the rich and poor may be at least as important as the *quantity* of care delivered. If the poor tend to visit facilities that are less well-equipped or receive care from providers who exert less effort, then they will be doubly penalized. Ultimately, of course, we are interested in these inequalities because they may lead to inequalities in actual health outcomes. There is evidence that this is indeed the case in ECA (World Bank 2012b).

In sum, empirical evidence suggests that households in about half of ECA's countries are spending significantly more on health, and with greater variation, than counterparts in EU-15 countries. A large share of this OOP spending is on drugs. Not surprisingly, indicators of catastrophic and impoverishing OOP payments are worse in countries that rely heavily on OOP spending for health financing. Catastrophic spending is slightly more common among higher socioeconomic groups, while the main consequence of weak financial protection for lower socioeconomic groups is forgone care, as reflected in higher inequality in utilization. Policies aimed at improving financial protection should be measured and monitored closely, and there is scope for improving current practices in this regard (box 4.2).

While over-reliance on OOP spending is a major challenge in about half the countries in ECA, in many of the others there is a significant health equity agenda related to the Roma population. Box 4.3 provides a summary of recent research on this issue.

BOX 4.2

Better Measurement of OOP Spending Will Help Inform Policies to Improve Financial Protection

Most ECA countries have long-standing traditions of collecting household budget survey (HBS) data on a regular (quarterly or annual) basis. These serve an invaluable role in assessing general economic conditions, measuring trends in living standards and poverty, monitoring government spending programs, and other purposes. They also provide an excellent opportunity for measuring and monitoring out-of-pocket payments for health, including for different socioeconomic groups. This potential is achieved in some countries, but in others there is substantial scope for improvement.

Estimating out-of-pocket payments through household surveys can be challenging. Rare events such as hospitalizations are more easily captured through longer recall periods, whereas more regular occurrences such as drug purchases or clinic visits are better addressed over shorter periods to reduce recall bias. Different recall periods can result in significantly different results (Das, Hammer, and Sanchez-Paramo 2012). Better information can often be achieved using contextual questions related to specific visits, which also allows for the collection of utilization data. But this requires care. Survey respondents may be asked about their last visit to a health care provider and the associated expenditures, often restricted to a certain time frame such as the past month. However, those who are sick, especially with a chronic illness, may make several visits during that period and often to more than one provider, with expenditures at each stage. Also, surveys may ask about drug purchases in association with a provider visit, whereas spending may occur in isolation from a health care episode (for example, self-treatment).

For these reasons, guidelines for health modules tend to recommend a more thorough survey to capture all visits and multiple recall periods, depending on the type of service—for example, one month for outpatient care and 12 months for inpatient care (Gertler, Rose, and Glewwe 2000). But an extensive health module may not be feasible in the context of a general consumption expenditure survey. The challenge is to combine the benefits of a detailed health module in a one-time stand-alone survey with the regular, institutionalized household budget surveys that yield robust information about living standards from consumption modules, thereby allowing for analysis of health-related indicators by socioeconomic status.

There is considerable empirical evidence that OOP is underestimated by many surveys. Estimates of health spending based on Living Standards Measurements Surveys (LSMS) tend to be much higher than household budget survey estimates (World Bank 2005). An analysis of differences between OOP estimates in surveys with both a detailed health module and a small number of health questions within a standard consumption module found that the latter tends to capture only between a quarter and a half of the health spending as the full health module. Of course, general household spending is also underestimated in survey data, but the problem appears to be notably more acute in the case of health expenditures (World Bank 2005). Methodological work is ongoing on this issue (Rannan-Eliya and Lorenzoni 2010; Heijink et al. 2011).

BOX 4.3

Significant Gaps in Roma Health in Central and Eastern Europe

In 2011, a Roma Regional Survey (RRS) was undertaken across six countries of Central and Eastern Europe: Bulgaria, the Czech Republic, Hungary, the former Yugoslav Republic of Macedonia, Romania, and the Slovak Republic. The objective was to collect information on the health status, access to public health infrastructure, and health care utilization of Roma populations in the region and to compare that with both their respective national averages and the non-Roma communities living nearby. Many smaller-scale studies have documented poor health outcomes among the Roma, showing a significant disadvantage in life expectancy, as well as infant and child mortality. The RRS adds to this body of evidence by describing the health-related vulnerabilities of the Roma populations across several dimensions from a broader comparative perspective both within and across the six countries surveyed (UNDP, World Bank, and EC 2011).

The findings confirm that the Roma are in poor health, not just compared to the (richer) general populations of the countries in which they reside, but in many respects even relative to non-Roma who live in the same communities. When asked to rate their own health, many Roma report that they are in poor health, while chronic disease estimates reveal a burden comparable to that among general populations, a surprising finding given that the Roma populations are considerably younger. Comprehensive regional data on infectious disease are not available for the Roma and were not collected in the survey, but smaller-scale studies show that the infectious disease burden is significant among the Roma. Roma of higher socioeconomic status are also in better health.

Findings from the RRS also show that access to public health goods remains very poor among the Roma across the six countries. While those in the Czech Republic and Hungary do have better access to most public health goods such as piped drinking water, waste management systems, and sanitation, coverage is far from adequate among most Roma households in vulnerable communities, especially those in Bulgaria and Romania. Vaccination rates are very low, with the vast majority of children not having received even at least one dose of each of the recommended vaccines. Even in countries with a relatively high overall coverage of vaccinations, such as the Czech Republic and Hungary, the vulnerable Roma were at a sizable disadvantage relative to their non-Roma neighbors.

Given the lower health status of the Roma, do they access the services they need through national health systems? Evidence from the RRS reveals that a large fraction of Roma forgo health care when needed, that utilization of outpatient services is positively correlated with socioeconomic status, and that the cost of health services is one of the most frequently cited barriers to access. The rate of forgone care is significantly lower among their non-Roma neighbors, and while this difference is in large part explained by the lower socioeconomic status of the Roma, a significant fraction of the Roma disadvantage remains unexplained

continued

BOX 4.3 *continued*

(see figure B.4.3.1). The rate of forgone care is highest in Bulgaria, which is also the country with the largest gap between the Roma and their non-Roma neighbors. In all other countries, forgone care was at least 30 percent, and the Roma disadvantage was sizable in the Czech Republic, the Slovak Republic, and Hungary. In the area of reproductive health, the RRS revealed that most Roma women deliver in hospitals, but further data collection is required to provide a more complete picture of services accessed during the antenatal and postnatal stages, as well as their quality.

FIGURE B4.3.1

Barriers to Access Are Significant among the Roma

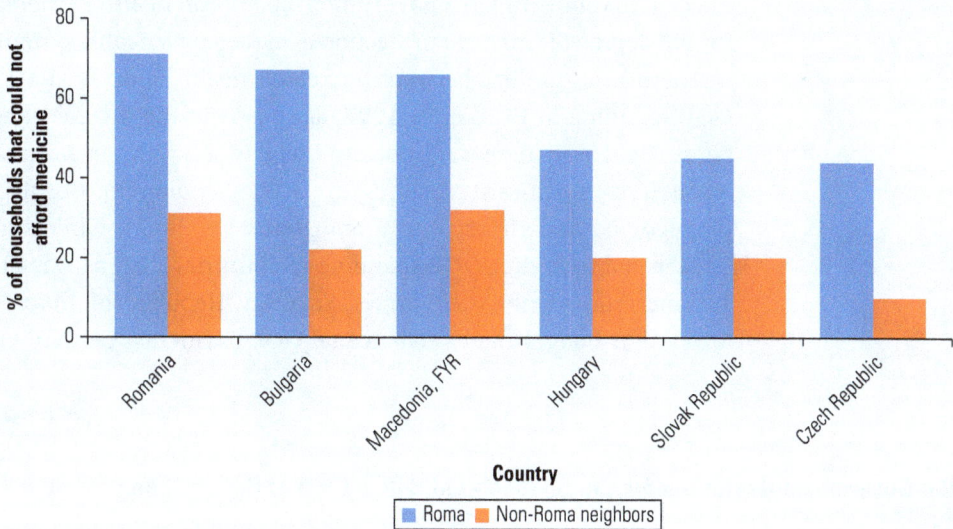

Source: UNDP, World Bank, and EC 2011.
Note: Figure shows rate of forgone care among the Roma population and their non-Roma neighbors.

Better Financial Protection Depends on Adequate Health Budgets and Control of Rent Seeking

Improving financial protection requires some understanding of the causes behind the stylized facts highlighted in the previous section. In this section, we focus on three main issues: the level of government spending, informal payments to providers, and pharmaceutical expenditures. For each, we also consider potential policy solutions. A key message is that an adequate government health budget is a necessary but not sufficient condition for achieving financial protection. Supply-side measures are also important.

More Public Spending Is Sometimes Needed to Improve Financial Protection

The ratio of government health spending to gross domestic product (GDP) is an important determinant of the share of total health expenditures financed out of pocket. The first panel of figure 4.6 shows the strong association between these two indicators across the region based on 2010 data. That association also holds true at the global level. Additional public resources for health have been identified as a key pillar in worldwide efforts to achieve universal coverage (WHO 2010). As shown in the previous section, overall reliance on OOP spending is positively correlated with the incidence of catastrophic health expenditures and inequality of utilization. Figures 4.6 and 4.7 indicate that how much a government spends on health matters a lot for the degree of financial protection achieved by a health system.

There is also a link between increased health budgets and lower OOP spending in ECA since 1997, as shown in the second panel in figure 4.6. Large increases in health budgets between 1997 and 2010 resulted in significant declines in OOP spending in Bosnia and Herzegovina and Turkey (Aran and Hentschel 2012), while smaller budgets led to higher OOP spending in countries such as Russia and Turkmenistan. Only the Former Yugoslav Republic of Macedonia lowered its budget *and* its reliance on OOP payments. Certainly most

FIGURE 4.6

Smaller Government Health Budgets Are Associated with a Greater Reliance on OOP Spending

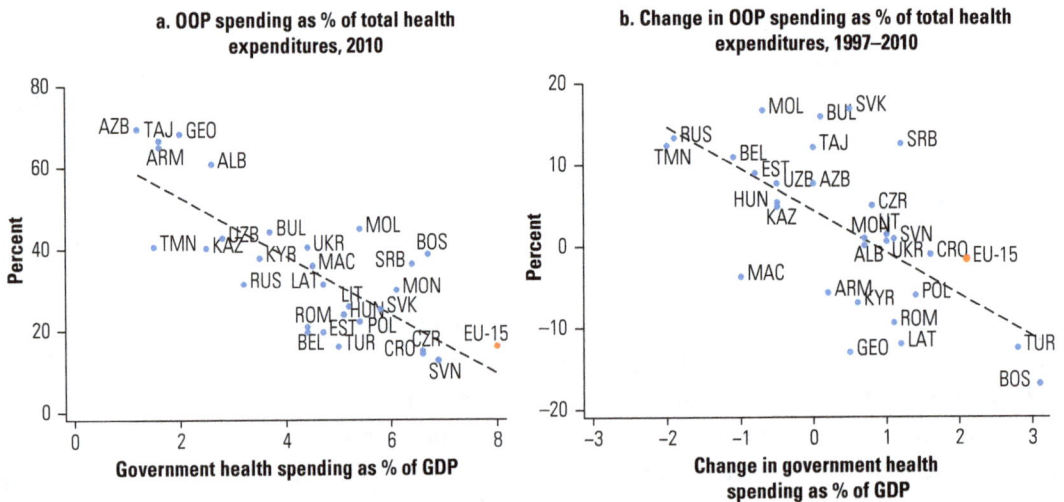

a. OOP spending as % of total health expenditures, 2010

b. Change in OOP spending as % of total health expenditures, 1997–2010

Source: WHO 2012.

Note: Figure shows link between government spending and out-of-pocket spending on health care for countries in Europe and Central Asia and the EU-15, 1997–2010. OOP = out of pocket.

FIGURE 4.7

Larger Government Health Budgets Are Associated with Better Financial Protection and Equity

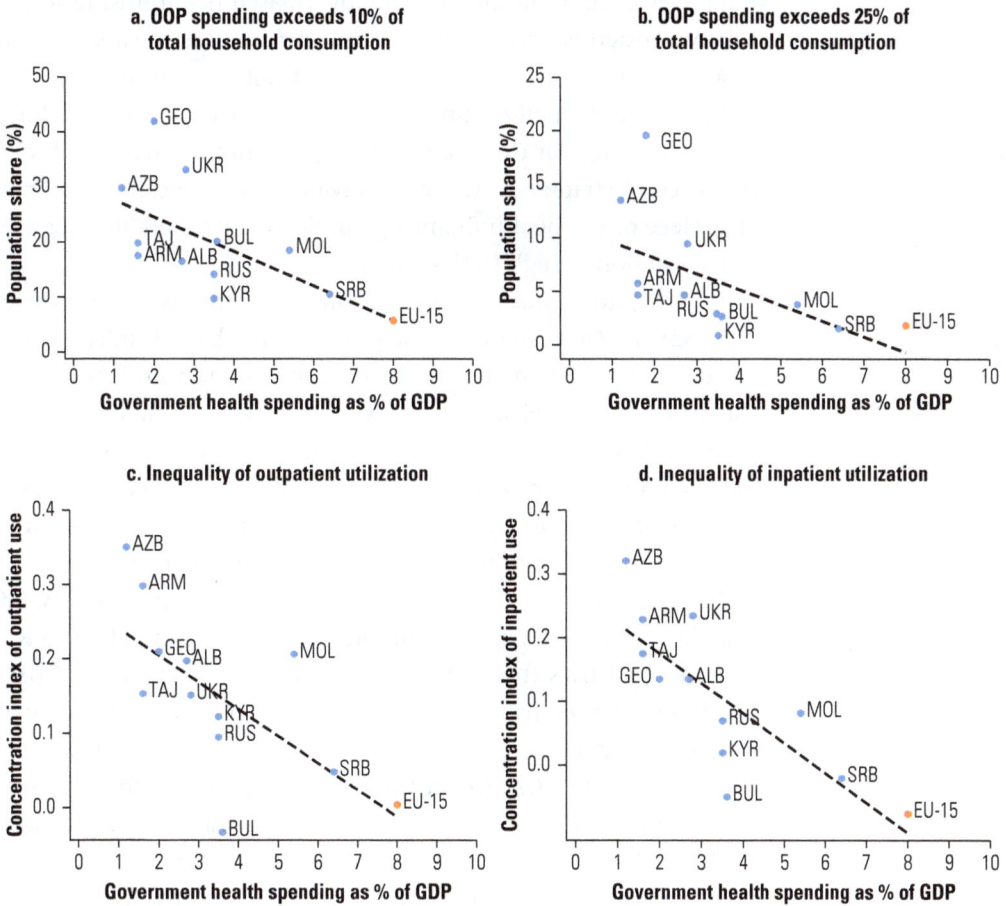

a. OOP spending exceeds 10% of total household consumption

(Population share (%) vs Government health spending as % of GDP)

b. OOP spending exceeds 25% of total household consumption

(Population share (%) vs Government health spending as % of GDP)

c. Inequality of outpatient utilization

(Concentration index of outpatient use vs Government health spending as % of GDP)

d. Inequality of inpatient utilization

(Concentration index of inpatient use vs Government health spending as % of GDP)

Source: Ali and Smith 2012.
Note: OOP = out of pocket; GDP = gross domestic product.

health budgets have increased in real terms due to strong economic growth over this period, but this growth also triggers greater demand for services. Nevertheless, there is significant variation in OOP trends in countries with similar budgetary trajectories, indicating that increased spending is not the only factor, as discussed below.

The close relationship between public spending and OOP spending shown in figure 4.6 reflects the fact that private insurance—that is, nongovernment, non-OOP health spending—almost never accounts for more than 10 percent of total health expenditure around the world, as indicated by national health accounts data (WHO 2012). The few exceptions are either high-income countries, where supplementary private insurance covers about 10–15 percent of total health spending, or middle-income countries with high rates of income inequality, where the better-off have "opted out" of an underfunded public sector and into private employer-based health insurance. The relative insignificance of private insurance as a means of health finance worldwide reflects both market failure (particularly in the individual and small-group markets that prevail outside the formal sector) and popular expectations for a prominent government role as discussed in chapter 2. Although private insurance can be an important piece of the health financing puzzle, it is unlikely to offer a systemic solution to high OOP spending.

In brief, total health financing in a country is largely divided between an OOP share and a government-share funded through general taxes or mandatory contributions. Both in ECA and around the world, the total level of expenditure typically falls in a range between 5 and 10 percent of GDP, albeit somewhat more in richer, older countries and somewhat less in poorer, younger nations. In effect, regardless of the public-private mix, there is demand everywhere to spend a nonnegligible share of income on health.

The bottom line is that if government health spending is low, OOP spending for health will be a burden for many household budgets. As a result, countries that spend little more than 2 percent of GDP on health will generally have poor indicators of financial protection, as is true of Albania, Armenia, Azerbaijan, Georgia, Tajikistan, and Turkmenistan in ECA. Government spending on health may be low either because the overall budget is small or because the allocation to health within the existing fiscal envelope is low. The reason will help identify where to find additional resources for health. The deeper question of why some countries allocate more government spending to health than others was touched on in box 2.3 on the politics of health spending. Weak financial protection is also probably one of the factors that helps explain why health was the top choice for additional government spending by survey respondents in so many ECA countries, as highlighted in chapter 2.

To underline the link between government spending and financial protection, figure 4.7 shows the correlation between the indicators introduced earlier and government health spending as a share of GDP. It is noteworthy that financing levels are more predictive of financial protection in a country than specific aspects of health system design, such as whether there is a national health service model, a single insurance fund, or multiple insurers. This topic is discussed in more detail in chapter 6.

Thus, one aspect of the policy agenda for countries with very low spending levels will be to increase health budgets to improve financial protection. Of course, this increase will need to happen gradually and in line with fiscal constraints. How to spend a larger resource envelope to improve financial protection will vary from country to country. Some might add basic drugs, and preferably generics, to the benefit package. Others will need to make higher general budget transfers to cover the population groups outside the formal social security system. Yet others might require higher salaries for underpaid medical staff to deter informal payments. Historically, medical salaries have been below average national incomes in many ECA countries (Rechel and McKee 2009). In Azerbaijan, for example, the average doctor's salary is about twice the minimum wage, whereas doctors in OECD countries typically earn salaries that are three times higher than the *average* wage (Fujisawa and Lafortune 2008). Where salaries are not directly paid, reimbursement prices for services to ensure cost recovery will be required.

In a best-case scenario, an additional dollar of government health spending can reduce OOP spending by a greater amount because of the lower prices enabled by stronger purchasing power (including by reducing rent seeking). But this reduction is by no means guaranteed, as discussed below. Analysis of current OOP patterns—who is paying, for what, and to whom—will help inform policy makers how to ensure that increased budgets translate into better financial protection.

Special effort should be made to ensure that improvements in financial protection and access to care benefit the poorest first, through targeted health programs. Better-off households typically have more options for obtaining health coverage and are more resilient in the face of unexpected medical bills. But the poor and near-poor are much more vulnerable. Georgia offers a successful example of using a proxy means test to target additional health resources to the poor, as discussed in box 4.4.

But More Spending Is Not Always the Answer

While additional government health spending can help reduce reliance on OOP spending and thereby improve financial protection indicators, that reduction is by no means certain and will depend in part on how the spending is distributed across people and services. Indeed, figures 4.6 and 4.7 indicate significant variation in OOP reliance and financial protection indicators at similar levels of public spending. Some of this variation may reflect exogenous factors such as a country's age profile or income level, but in other cases there is scope for doing better through improved policies.

BOX 4.4

Targeting Spending to Reduce OOP Payments among the Poor: Georgia's Medical Insurance Program

Georgia's Medical Insurance Program (MIP) for the poor was introduced in 2007 and offers a comprehensive benefit package to eligible households. Most emergency outpatient care and planned or emergency inpatient care are included, with few coverage limits and no copayments. As of 2012, most of the non-MIP population had access to only a very basic package with significant copayments, a lack of clear definitions, chronic underfunding, and widespread informal payments. Eligibility for the MIP is determined by a proxy means test that includes over 100 indicators and is administered by the Social Services Agency to any household that applies (about 40 percent of the population has applied). The state budget covers all households up to a score of 70,000, while two regions, Adjara and Tbilisi, also cover households with scores between 70,000 and 100,000. As of 2011, the MIP covered 900,000 beneficiaries—about 20 percent of the population—and had a budget of about 0.6 percent of GDP, or somewhat less than half the state health budget.

To assess the impact of the MIP on key outcomes of interest, an evaluation comparing those just above and just below the eligibility threshold was carried out in 2008–09 (Bauhoff, Hotchkiss, and Smith 2011). Figure B4.4.1 shows the significant impact of the MIP on out-of-pocket expenditures for health care. For outpatient care in Adjara and Tbilisi, and inpatient care in all regions, MIP beneficiaries pay approximately 50 percent less than nonbeneficiaries (there is no statistically significant difference for outpatient care in the regions with a cutoff score of 70,000). The survey also found that MIP beneficiaries were more likely to report receiving free or reduced-price care because of insurance and less likely to report that they could not pay the costs of care out of their usual income. Together, these findings indicate that the MIP has made a major contribution to reducing out-of-pocket spending among its beneficiaries and is therefore achieving one of its key program goals. The survey results also indicated, however, that the program has not had any impact on utilization. A separate study based on nationally representative data found no significant change in the use of care by socioeconomic quintile between 2007 and 2010 (Ward 2010). The main reason why out-of-pocket spending has not fallen to zero among MIP members is that drug expenditures are, for the most part, excluded from the benefit package. However, some respondents also reported paying for certain services that are supposed to be covered by the MIP, indicating that informal payments may persist and that there is scope for improving knowledge of the benefit package.

The impact of a program may be different during its first two years of existence from what it is after 5 or 10 years, and thus continued monitoring will be important. Nationally, Georgia's financial protection indicators are among the weakest in ECA, and thus much progress remains to be made. Indeed, additional measures were under consideration by 2013. But the explicit targeting component of the MIP offers an example of how to prioritize additional spending within an expanded health budget.

continued

BOX 4.4 *continued*

FIGURE B4.4.1

Georgia's MIP Has Reduced OOP among the Poor

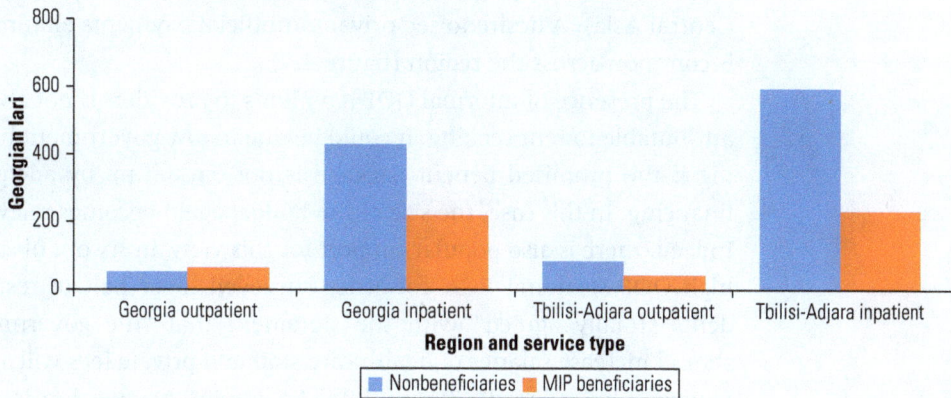

Source: Bauhoff, Hotchkiss, and Smith 2011.
Note: Figure shows OOP cost per episode. OOP = out of pocket; lari = Georgian currency; MIP = Medical Insurance Program.

Although global evidence also lends support to the view that "more money" or "coverage" can help, they do not always translate into improved financial protection (Wagstaff 2008). An expansion of government-funded health care (irrespective of the funding model) will tend to increase the quantity of care received, which will put upward pressure on OOP spending when the generosity of coverage is less than 100 percent, as found in China and Vietnam. Copayments, deductibles, reimbursement ceilings, and, perhaps most important, excluded items such as drugs will result in *more* OOP spending as service use increases.

The Challenge of Informal Payments: Addressing Rent Seeking by Providers

An important reason why more government spending does not necessarily translate into better financial protection is due to rent seeking by providers of health care, another major cause of high OOP spending. Rent seeking may take the form of either higher prices or unnecessary services and is rooted in the market power and informational advantages of providers as discussed earlier. Overprovision is discussed further in chapter 5; the focus here is on informal payments.

It is often difficult to properly measure and monitor informal OOP spending, precisely because it takes place unofficially, behind closed doors. But anecdotal evidence is abundant. The Life in Transition Survey, implemented in 29 ECA countries, found that unofficial payments are common in many (figure 4.8). When the sample is restricted to those who work as medical professionals, the reported frequency is only slightly lower (with the exception of Central Asia). A desire to see private unofficial payments eliminated is common across the region (figure 4.9).

The presence of informal OOP payments to providers is not always attributable to rent seeking. It could be due to low government funding if the promised benefit package is not backed up by adequate financing. In this case, the size of the budget again becomes relevant. Indeed, there is also popular support for this view. In six out of seven high-OOP-spending ECA countries surveyed, over half of respondents "totally agreed" with the statement that "the government should increase salaries of health care staff and private fees will automatically be reduced" (figure 4.9). An important question is thus whether informal payments reflect cost recovery or rent seeking. But answering this question can raise issues about appropriate pay for medical workers and the efficiency of medical care provision.

The main causes of informal payments are complex and have been the focus of several reviews (Ensor 2004; Lewis 2007; Rechel

FIGURE 4.8

Unofficial Payments for Medical Care Are Widely Acknowledged

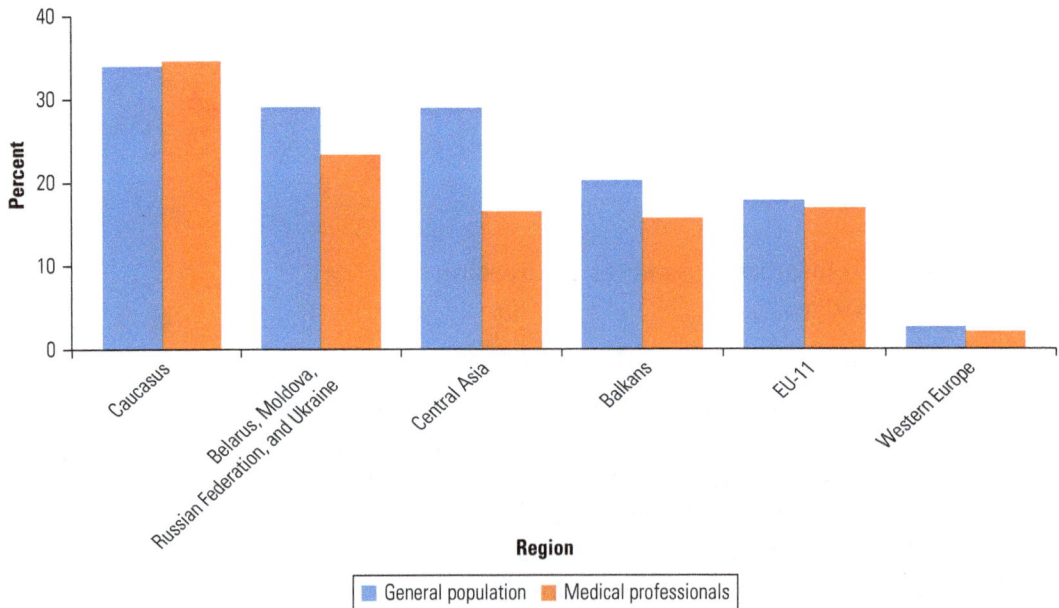

Source: EBRD 2010.
Note: Figure shows frequency of unofficial payments (percentage of respondents saying "usually" or "always").

FIGURE 4.9

Attitudes toward Unofficial Payments in ECA Highlight the Need for a Policy Response

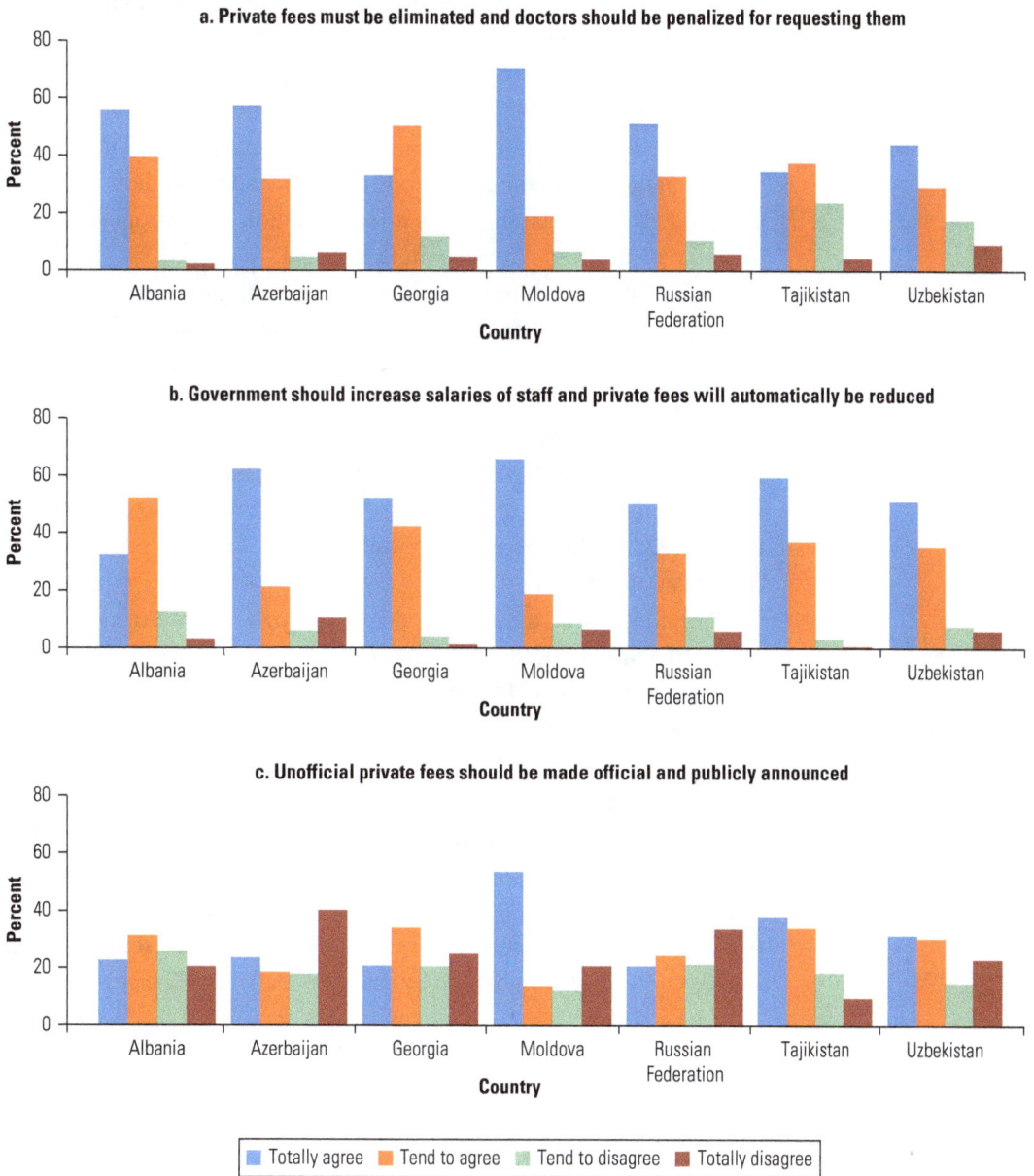

a. Private fees must be eliminated and doctors should be penalized for requesting them

b. Government should increase salaries of staff and private fees will automatically be reduced

c. Unofficial private fees should be made official and publicly announced

■ Totally agree ■ Tend to agree ■ Tend to disagree ■ Totally disagree

Source: World Bank 2012a.
Note: ECA = Europe and Central Asia.

and McKee 2009). They include low remuneration of staff, weak regulatory and accountability structures, underfunded and unclear benefit packages and exemption policies, and overcapacity. Hospital physicians tend to be the main participants. Long-standing traditions of gift giving are also a factor. In addition to the problems associated with formal OOP payments, including that they are regressive, unofficial payments also typically result in forgone tax revenues.

Various potential solutions exist for addressing informal payments. They can be made into official fees (as in the Kyrgyz Republic), with the consequent transparency and predictability helping to reduce rent seeking by providers. However, this measure will tend to be unpopular with the public (figure 4.9). The enforcement of regulation, potentially including measures to penalize medical staff for charging informal payments, is another option. The support of professional associations can help in this regard.

Accountability of providers can also be strengthened by enlisting patients in the fight against informal payments, especially through information, transparency, and grievance redress mechanisms. The Armenia case study in box 4.5 offers an example. A survey of institutional characteristics across health systems in ECA (discussed further in chapter 6) found that they have fewer accountability mechanisms— such as a patient desk at hospitals to register complaints or a national ombudsman with specific responsibilities for health care—than in OECD countries.

Ultimately, if corruption is endemic throughout government, then efforts to address unofficial payments for health care are likely to meet with limited success. In some ECA countries, doctors may charge unofficial fees to patients because they must pay the head doctor of the hospital for the privilege of practicing there, and the head doctor in turn may be expected to pay hospital ownership (for example, municipal, district, or national governments) for the right to retain his or her position. Health systems generate significant revenue streams that offer a rent-seeking opportunity for individuals well beyond hospital or clinic walls. To overcome informal payments in this setting, broad multisectoral strategies backed by strong leadership will be essential.

Rent Seeking Also Matters for Drugs

A particularly important cause of high out-of-pocket spending is expenditures on pharmaceuticals, which account for over half of total OOP payments in several countries, as noted earlier. To a significant extent, these high costs result from the low drug coverage provided by benefit packages in ECA. Third-party payers cover almost 70 percent of drug spending in OECD countries, while in ECA, this ratio is usually well under half, and often as little as 10 percent. Overconsumption may also be a problem, which can be driven by the demand- or by the supply-side, or by both. Regulatory issues are important, such as a lack of rational prescribing patterns.

BOX 4.5

Reducing Informal Payments with Accountability: Armenia's Maternity Voucher Program

For many years, delivering a child in Armenia was a costly proposition, despite being officially free. Anecdotes of new mothers trying to "escape" from hospitals to avoid high informal payments abounded. In 2008, a new policy initiative aimed to address this problem. It included three main components. First, costing evidence suggested that reimbursement rates for deliveries were inadequate, covering only half the actual costs. Thus, prices paid to hospitals were sharply increased. But this alone would not guarantee an end to informal payments. The second measure was stronger regulation of how the additional funds should be allocated within hospitals—in particular, to ensure a fair distribution between frontline medical staff (doctors and nurses) and hospital management, who were known to extract significant payments from staff. The third measure sought to ensure that patients were well informed about the new policy and that they had avenues for recourse if needed. For this purpose, all expectant mothers received a voucher for delivery during antenatal care, clearly stating that absolutely no payment was required and providing telephone hotline numbers in case of problems.

Figure B4.5.1 shows the impact of this initiative on reported OOP payments for child deliveries, with a steep decline soon after the reform was launched in July 2008. The proportion of new mothers who paid nothing increased sharply at the same time. Phone calls to the hotline were relatively frequent in the first two months of the reform, prompting follow-up by the Ministry of Health with hospitals. Initially a large proportion of the hotline calls were complaints, while the rest were seeking information. Soon the complaint calls diminished in number, suggesting that the reform was working. By November 2008, no complaints were received by the hotline. We cannot be certain that informal payments did not resurface for other (nonmaternity) services, but the policy is being expanded and will require continued monitoring.

FIGURE B4.5.1

Armenia's Maternity Voucher Program Has Had a Large Impact on Informal Payments

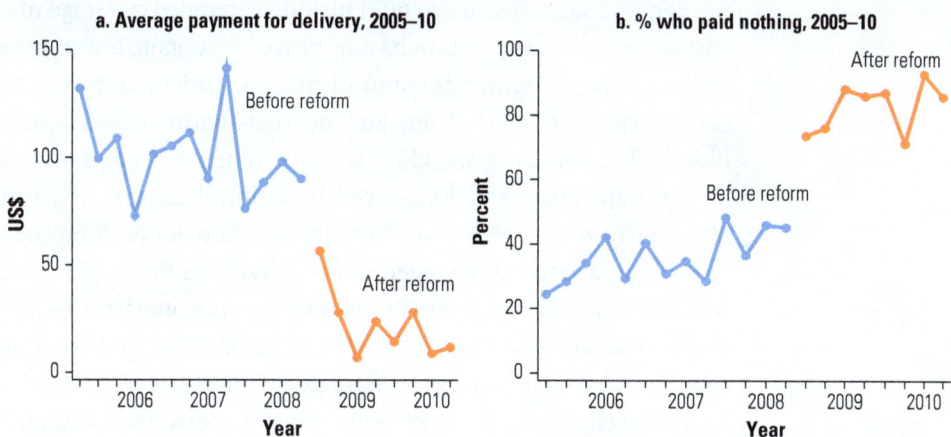

Source: World Bank 2011.

Various forms of rent seeking pervade the pharmaceutical sector. Some of this behavior may include direct payments to doctors by pharmaceutical agents to promote their own drugs or hospitals that reap gains from their own pharmacy sales. But high retail prices are also a big part of the story, in part due to a lack of availability of generic drugs. Pharmacy surveys in Armenia and Georgia, for example, have found that generic equivalents for a large number of common drugs were available in fewer than half the pharmacies visited. Also, the import, wholesale, distribution, and retail networks for pharmaceutical products can be subject to significant market concentration. All EU countries (independently) regulate price margins for drugs, with combined wholesale and retail markups commonly around 30 percent. A study in Georgia in 2010 found the average combined wholesale and retail margins across a list of 50 common drugs were over 100 percent, while the average markup in the Czech Republic, Hungary, and Poland was between 25 and 35 percent for the same list of drugs (World Bank 2012c). Earlier work found that retail drug prices were twice as high as wholesale prices in Kazakhstan (Ensor and Savelyeva 1998).

Supply-side measures to reduce OOP spending on pharmaceuticals offer significant opportunities for improving financial protection. On the quantity side, the promotion of rational drug policies, such as treatment protocols and drug lists, is a key intervention in this respect. Stricter controls on drug promotion, marketing, education, and sponsorship gifts to doctors could also help. On the price side, promoting generic drugs can significantly lower overall spending levels (Cameron and Laing 2010). Direct regulation of pharmaceutical price markups, as is the case in most advanced countries, is another potential measure. This approach could include higher margins on cheaper generic drugs, thereby motivating more dispensing of generics. On the demand side, measures could include expanded coverage of drugs and subsequent use of purchasing power to obtain lower prices as well as influencing the demand of insured patients through higher cost sharing for brand drugs and no cost-sharing for generics. But ultimately, some drug spending is likely to be discretionary spending by the population and influenced by cultural factors, and thus an objective of zero OOP spending on drugs would not be appropriate.

Overall, a large policy agenda for improving financial protection remains in those ECA countries where key outcomes in this area are weak. Once adequate health budgets have been secured, for a significant share of OOP payments, stronger financial protection can best be achieved through supply-side interventions rather than with more money or expanded coverage.

References

Ali, R., and O. Smith. 2012. "Financial Protection and Equity in Europe and Central Asia." Draft. World Bank, Washington, DC.

Aran, M., and J. Hentschel. 2012. "Protection in Good and Bad Times? The Turkish Green Card Health Program." Policy Research Working Paper 6178, World Bank, Washington, DC.

Arrow, K. 1963. "Uncertainty and the Welfare Economics of Medical Care." *American Economic Review* 53 (5): 941–73.

Baicker, K., and D. Goldman. 2011. "Patient Cost-Sharing and Health Care Spending Growth." *Journal of Economic Perspectives* 25 (2): 47–68.

Baicker, K., S. Mullainathan, and J. Schwartzstein. 2012. "Behavioral Hazard in Health Insurance." NBER Working Paper 18468, National Bureau of Economic Research, Cambridge, MA.

Bauhoff, S., D. Hotchkiss, and O. Smith. 2011. "The Impact of Medical Insurance for the Poor in Georgia: A Regression Discontinuity Approach." *Health Economics* 20: 1362–78.

Belli, P., G. Gotsadze, and H. Shahriari. 2004. "Out-of-Pocket and Informal Payments in Health Sector: Evidence from Georgia." *Health Policy* 70 (1): 109–23.

Bredenkamp, C., M. Mendola, and M. Gragnolati. 2011. "Catastrophic and Impoverishing Effects of Health Expenditure: New Evidence from the Western Balkans." *Health Policy and Planning* 26 (4): 1–8.

Cameron, A., and R. Laing. 2010. "Cost Savings of Switching Private Sector Consumption from Originator Brand Medicines to Generic Equivalents." World Health Report Background Paper 35, World Health Organization, Geneva.

Chernew, M. E., A. B. Rosen, and A. M. Fendrick. 2007. "Value-Based Insurance Design." *Health Affairs* 26 (2): 195–203.

Chetty R., and A. Looney. 2006. "Consumption Smoothing and the Welfare Consequences of Social Insurance in Developing Economies." *Journal of Public Economics* 90: 2351–56.

———. 2007. "Income Risk and the Benefits of Social Insurance: Evidence from Indonesia and the United States." In *Fiscal Policy and Management in East Asia: NBER East Asia Seminar on Economics*, vol. 16, edited by T. Ito and A. Rose. Chicago: University of Chicago Press.

Das, J., J. Hammer, and C. Sanchez-Paramo. 2012. "The Impact of Recall Periods on Reported Morbidity and Health Seeking Behavior." *Journal of Development Economics* 98 (1): 76–88.

Deaton, A., and S. Zaidi. 2002. "Guidelines for Construction Consumption Aggregates for Welfare Analysis." LSMS Working Paper 135, Living Standards Measurement Survey, World Bank, Washington, DC.

Demirguc-Kunt, A., and L. Klapper. 2012. "Measuring Financial Inclusion: The Global Findex Database." Policy Research Working Paper 6025, World Bank, Washington, DC.

Ensor, T. 2004. "Informal Payments for Health Care in Transition Economies." *Social Science and Medicine* 58: 237–46.

Ensor T., and L. Savelyeva. 1998. "Informal Payments for Health Care in the Former Soviet Union: Some Evidence from Kazakhstan." *Health Policy and Planning* 13 (1): 41–49.

EBRD (European Bank for Reconstruction and Development). 2010. *Life in Transition Survey.* http://www.ebrd.com/pages/research/publications/special/transitionII.shtml.

Falkingham, J., B. Akkazieva, and A. Baschieri. 2010. "Trends in Out-of-Pocket Payments for Health Care in Kyrgyzstan, 2001–07." *Health Policy and Planning* 25: 427–36.

Flores, G., J. Krishnakumar, O. O'Donnell, and E. van Doorslaer. 2008. "Coping with Health Care Costs: Implications for the Measurement of Catastrophic Expenditures and Poverty." *Health Economics* 17: 1393–1412.

Fujisawa, R., and G. Lafortune. 2008. "The Remuneration of General Practitioners and Specialists in 14 OECD Countries: What Are the Factors Influencing Variations across Countries?" Health Working Paper 41, Organisation for Economic Co-operation and Development, Paris.

Gertler, P., E. Rose, and P. Glewwe. 2000. "Health." In *Designing Household Survey Questionnaires for Developing Countries: Lessons from 15 years of the Living Standards Measurement Study*, edited by M. Grosh and P. Glewwe, 177–216. Washington, DC: World Bank.

Gertler P., and J. Gruber. 2002. "Insuring Consumption against Illness." *American Economic Review* 92 (1): 51–76.

Habicht, J., K. Xu, A. Couffinhal, and J. Kutzin. 2006. "Detecting Changes in Financial Protection: Creating Evidence for Policy in Estonia." *Health Policy Planning* 21 (6): 421–31.

Heijink, R., K. Xu, P. Saksena, and D. Evans. 2011. "Validity and Comparability of Out-of-Pocket Health Expenditure from Household Surveys: A Review of the Literature and Current Survey Instruments." WHO Health System Financing Discussion Paper 1, World Health Organization, Geneva.

Lambrelli, D., and O. O'Donnell. 2009. "The Large Burden of Direct Payments for Health in Greece in Comparison with other European Countries." In *Life 50+: Health, Ageing and Pensions in Greece and Europe,* edited by A. Lyberaki, P. Tinios, and T. Filalithis. Athens: Kritiki.

Lewis, M. 2007. "Informal Payments and the Financing of Health Care in Developing and Transition Countries." *Health Affairs* 26 (4): 984–97.

Liebman, J., and R. Zeckhauser. 2008. "Simple Humans, Complex Insurance, Subtle Subsidies." NBER Working Paper 14330, National Bureau of Economic Research, Cambridge, MA.

Manning, W., J. Newhouse, N. Duan, E. Keeler, A. Leibowitz, and S. Marquis. 1987. "Health Insurance and the Demand for Medical Care: Evidence from a Randomized Experiment." *American Economic Review* 77 (3): 251–77.

O'Donnell, O., E. van Doorslaer, A. Wagstaff, and M. Lindelow. 2008. *Analyzing Health Equity Using Household Surveys: A Guide to Techniques and Their Implementation.* Washington, DC: World Bank.

OECD (Organisation for Economic Co-operation and Development). 2011. *Health at a Glance 2011.* Paris: Organisation for Economic Co-operation and Development.

Pauly, M. V. 1968. "The Economics of Moral Hazard: Comment." *American Economic Review* 58 (3): 531–37.

Rannan-Eliya, R. P., and L. Lorenzoni. 2010. "Guidelines for Improving the Comparability and Availability of Private Health Expenditures under the System of Health Accounts Framework." OECD Health Working Paper 52, Organisation for Economic Co-operation and Development, Paris.

Rechel, B., and M. McKee. 2009. "Health Reform in Central and Eastern Europe and the Former Soviet Union." *Lancet* 374: 1186–95.

Tomini, S., and T. Packard. 2011. "Are Health Care Payments in Albania Catastrophic? Evidence from ALSMS 2002, 2005, and 2008." UNU Merit Working Paper 19, United Nations University, Maastricht.

Townsend, R. 1995. "Consumption Insurance: An Evaluation of Risk-Bearing Systems in Low-Income Economies." *Journal of Economic Perspectives* 9 (3): 83–102.

UNDP (United Nations Development Programme), World Bank, and EC (European Commission). 2011. *Regional Roma Survey.* Draft. United Nations Development Programme, World Bank, and European Commission.

van Doorslaer, E., O. O'Donnell, R. P. Raannan-Eliya, A. Somanathan, S. R. Adhikari, C. C. Garg, et al. 2006. "Effect of Payments for Health Care on Poverty Estimates in 11 Countries in Asia: An Analysis of Household Survey Data." *Lancet* 368: 1357–64.

———. 2007. "Catastrophic Payments for Health Care in Asia." *Health Economics* 16 (11): 1159–84.

van Doorslaer, E., X. Koolman, and A. M. Jones. 2004. "Explaining Income-Related Inequalities in Doctor Utilization in Europe." *Health Economics* 13: 629–47.

van Doorslaer, E., and C. Masseria. 2004. "Income-Related Inequality in the Use of Medical Care in 21 OECD Countries." OECD Health Working Paper 14, Organisation for Economic Co-operation and Development, Paris.

Wagstaff, A. 2008. "Measuring Financial Protection." Policy Research Working Paper 4554, World Bank, Washington, DC.

Ward, P. 2010. Georgia Health Utilization and Expenditure Survey. Draft. Oxford.

Waters, H., J. Hobart, C. B. Forrest, K. K. Siemens, P. M. Pittman, A. Murthy, et al. 2008. "Health Insurance Coverage in Central and Eastern Europe: Trends and Challenges." *Health Affairs* 27 (2): 478–86, http://content. healthaffairs.org/content/27/2/478.abstract.

World Bank. 2005. *Growth, Poverty, and Inequality in Eastern Europe and the Former Soviet Union.* Washington, DC: World Bank.

———. 2011. "Public Expenditure Review: Fiscal Consolidation and Recovery in Armenia." http://documents.worldbank.org/curated/en/2012/01 /16764733/fiscal-consolidation-recovery-armenia-impact-global-crisis -small-open-economy.

———. 2012a. "Findings from a Household Survey on Health in 6 ECA Countries." Draft. World Bank, Washington, DC.

———. 2012b. "Financial Protection and Equity Fact-Sheets for ECA." Washington, DC, World Bank.

_____. 2012c. "Georgia Public Expenditure Review: Managing Expenditure Pressures for Sustainability and Growth." http://documents.worldbank.org/curated/en/2012/11/17091988/georgia-managing-expenditure-pressures-sustainability-growth-public-expenditure-review.

WHO (World Health Organization). 2010. *World Health Report: The Path to Universal Coverage*. Geneva: WHO.

———. 2012. Global Health Expenditure Database, http://apps.who.int/nha/database.

Xu, K., P. Saksena, M. Jowett, C. Indikadahena, J. Kutzin, and D. Evans. 2010. "Exploring the Thresholds of Health Expenditure for Protection against Financial Risk." Background Paper 19, World Health Report 2010, World Health Organization, Geneva.

Zeckhauser, R. 1970. "Medical Insurance: A Case Study of the Tradeoff between Risk Spreading and Appropriate Incentives." *Journal of Economic Theory* 2 (1): 10–26.

CHAPTER 5

Improving Efficiency: Cutting the Fat

Key Messages

- Although health budgets have not grown as fast in ECA as in other regions, the efficiency of health spending is a major concern.

- While the growth rate of health budgets and their efficiency and fiscal sustainability are important considerations, ultimately, health spending should be judged by its costs and benefits.

- The social costs of government health budgets are the cost of revenue raising and the moral hazard loss due to excess consumption by the insured; the social benefits of health spending are the value of any health gains and the benefit of risk protection against high and unpredictable medical costs.

- Hospitals are a key source of waste, especially in CIS countries. Across ECA, pharmaceuticals are an additional major driver of excess costs.

- There are few easy answers to the efficiency agenda—some commonly cited proposals to improve efficiency have important drawbacks.

- A major challenge posed by the efficiency agenda is that while health systems often have a large amount of waste, at the same time they provide some very high value care, and the imperative is to find a way to cut one without cutting the other.

- Evidence suggests that health systems in advanced countries have provided high value for money on average but significant waste on the margin.

- A large part of the efficiency agenda is not about pursuing major systemic reforms but rather about understanding and addressing variation in outputs and outcomes by provider and service type.

The government health budget can create angst among fiscal policy makers like few other topics. It is often seen as wasteful and inefficient, and the tendency of health spending around the world to rise faster than per capita gross domestic product (GDP) is seen as a threat to fiscal sustainability and growth. Concerns about the efficiency of the health system are well grounded. But in previous chapters, we have also seen that health spending is a top priority of populations and voters across the region, that it can improve health outcomes, and that it can help protect households from financial risk and equalize access to care. How to manage these tensions is a key policy challenge for countries in Europe and Central Asia (ECA) and elsewhere.

Budget pressures in health sectors worldwide have received growing attention from both policy makers and international institutions in recent years (World Bank 2007; OECD 2009a, 2010; European Commission 2010; IMF 2012). Figure 5.1 shows government health spending as a share of GDP across ECA in 2010. As discussed in chapter 1, over the past decade or so, most countries in ECA have done a better job of keeping a lid on their health budgets than the countries in the EU-15 have done. Only 2 out of 29 countries had a larger percentage-point increase in health spending as a share of GDP than their Western European comparators, while only 5 had a larger increase as a share of the total government budget (see figure 1.4).

FIGURE 5.1

Government Health Spending in ECA, 2010

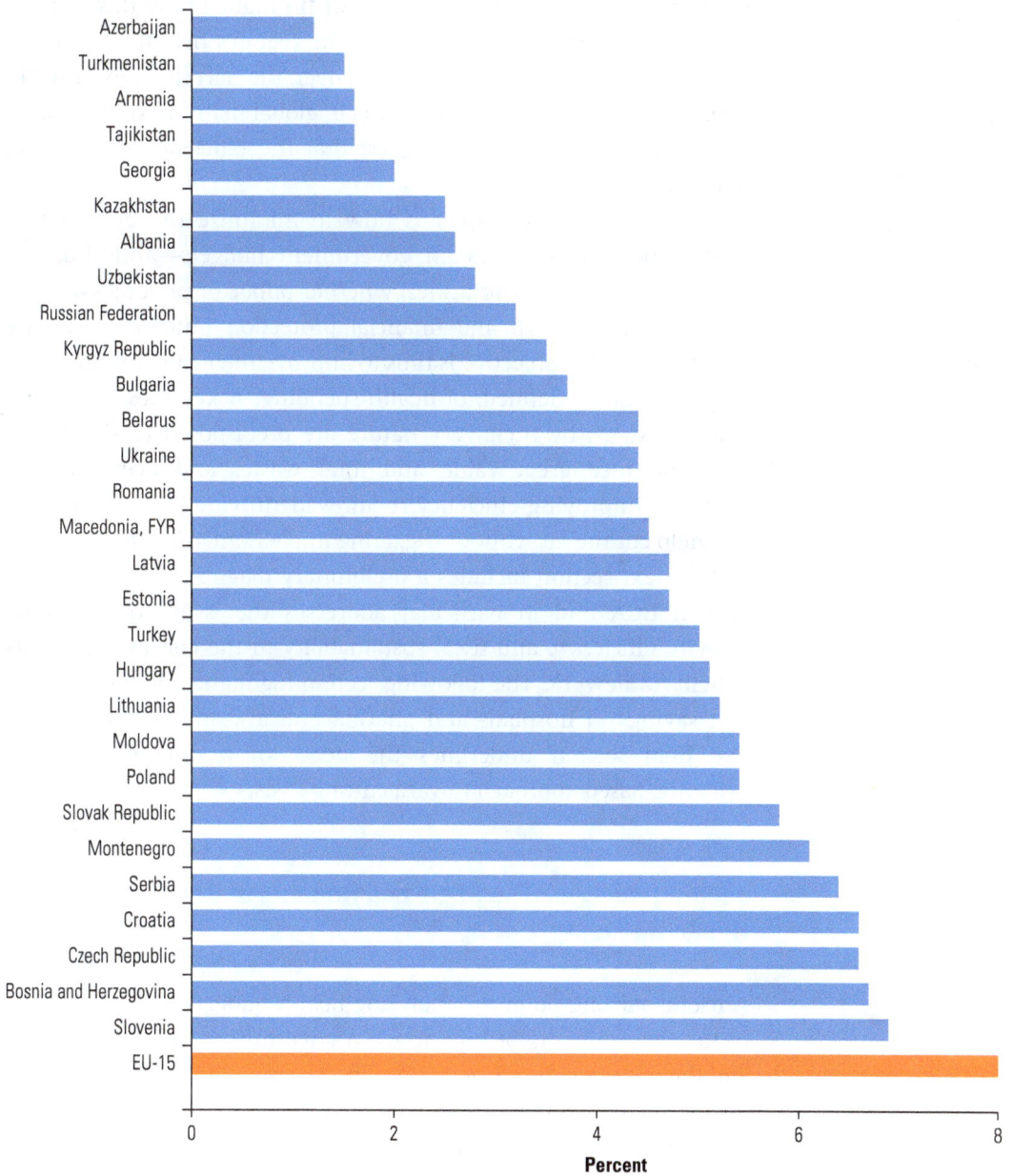

Source: WHO 2012a.
Note: Figure shows government health spending as percentage of GDP. ECA = Europe and Central Asia; GDP = gross domestic product.

The lack of convergence of ECA's health spending levels with those of the EU-15 is good news from a narrow fiscal perspective, but at least in some countries, it has probably come at the expense of better health and financial protection outcomes, as indicated in previous chapters. It is also true that much of ECA enjoyed robust economic growth for many years before the recent crisis, and thus the real value of spending increased significantly in many countries, even if its share of GDP was more stable. But no matter how this trend is interpreted, there is little doubt that the region's health systems are not as efficient as they could be. Moreover, the narratives explored in earlier chapters and the widespread global pattern of persistent growth in health spending suggest that the efficiency agenda will loom ever larger in the future.

The focus of this chapter is how to minimize the burden that health spending imposes on government budgets—and thus the crowding out of other priorities, whether public or private—without sacrificing the health and financial protection outcomes we care about. The policy objective is thus to improve the value for money, or *efficiency* broadly defined, of health spending. A key message is that health systems by their very nature are predisposed to simultaneously produce great value and total waste, and everything in between. Improving efficiency requires identifying instruments that will help cut the fat without triggering unpleasant side effects.

The next section includes a preliminary diagnosis of health budgets in ECA and in particular addresses the issues of spending, growth, efficiency, and fiscal sustainability in the context of a cost-benefit framework. The following section highlights the potential for cost savings in hospitals and pharmaceuticals, among other areas. The final section underlines the need for a discretionary and evidence-based approach toward cutting costs.

Judging Budgets: The Costs and Benefits of Government Health Spending

A useful starting point for analyzing health budgets is a brief survey of the determinants of how much a government spends on health and the growth rate, efficiency, and fiscal sustainability of that spending. These are sometimes all conflated into a single "problem"; but although related, they are conceptually distinct.

Diagnosing Health Spending Levels, Growth Rates, Efficiency, and Fiscal Sustainability

Around the world, almost all countries spend between 5 and 10 percent of total GDP on health (public and private), with richer and older countries at the higher end of this range and poorer, younger nations at the lower end. This total is divided for the most part between a government share and an out-of-pocket (OOP) share, due to the limitations of private voluntary pooling. Institutional and political factors also play a role in how much is spent. From a simpler accounting perspective, health spending can also be seen as price multiplied by quantity. In ECA, countries are scattered across the full range of spending levels.

The growth of health spending is largely due to four factors: rising incomes, aging populations, the expansion of insurance coverage, and the adoption of new technologies. Each matters individually, and they can also be mutually reinforcing. Of these, the most important has been technological change. Fifty years ago, there were few treatment options for a 65-year-old with coronary heart disease. Today, thanks to new technology, a lot can be done. The same is true of many other diseases. Underlying all four determinants is another factor: preferences. As people grow richer, the relative importance of living long, healthy lives grows steadily and with it the willingness to forgo other consumption. As noted, the average growth of health spending in ECA over the past 15 years has been relatively low by global standards, but there is no guarantee that this trend will continue.

The contribution of aging in particular to rising health spending has not been as large as is sometimes believed. While per capita health spending on the elderly is roughly three times higher than on younger adults, demographic shifts happen too slowly to explain the large historical increases in overall health spending. In the future, aging may account for about one-quarter of growth in health spending in ECA if the experience of advanced countries is repeated. Since the aging process is essentially "locked in" while the other drivers of health spending are amenable to some policy intervention, rising health expenditures do not need to be seen as inevitable.

Addressing efficiency is a challenge for essentially every health system. In fact, several aspects of the health sector would appear to make it especially predisposed to inefficiency. Market failures in health financing require a prominent role for government, including through taxation, with resulting distortions to economic behavior. The uncertainty of health care needs brings us into the "second-best" world of a trade-off between risk pooling and moral hazard, in which the absence of insurance is itself a form of inefficiency. Third-party purchasing blunts the price signal on both the supply and the demand side. Many of the suppliers of medical care, such as hospitals, doctors, and pharmaceutical companies, also have significant market power that can result in large rents. And finally, due to the highly individualized and discretionary nature of health care, it is difficult to monitor effort and quality in its provision, which poses a challenge for contracting out.

But while it is easy to enumerate these sources of inefficiency, it is far harder to overcome them. Nor is the measurement of efficiency straightforward, particularly when we try to move from outputs (for example, number of hospital admissions) to outcomes (mortality rates, for instance). How do we know if a particular procedure was necessary or not? If a patient's condition takes a turn for the better (worse), was it because of the care provided or just the underlying disease taking its course? Common techniques for measuring efficiency are problematic and should be approached with caution (Newhouse 1994; Hollingsworth 2008). On the system level, it is easier to identify static inefficiency at any point in time, but it is more difficult to say whether it is getting better or worse over time (Chernew and Newhouse 2012).

Fiscal sustainability is a much broader issue, embracing taxation, debt, and other sectoral expenditure policies and is not readily addressed on a sector-by-sector basis. In many countries in ECA, health is the second-largest spending category, albeit a distant second behind pension spending, and thus it has a large impact on the government's fiscal position. Clearly, the trend whereby growth in health spending exceeds overall economic growth cannot go on forever. But the point at which health expenditures become "too much" may be very high, since, as we saw in chapter 2, the trade-off between health and other goods will increasingly favor health as countries grow richer. For example, it has been argued that the *optimal* health share of total GDP in the United States may exceed 30 percent by 2050 (Hall and Jones 2007). But assessing fiscal sustainability in all its dimensions is beyond the scope of this report.

If the goal of policy were to limit government health expenditure to some target level, the solution would be relatively easy. For example, hard spending caps could be imposed on all facilities, above which no reimbursements would be made. But improving welfare is an altogether more difficult task, and thus a full assessment of health budgets must move beyond how much is spent and how efficient it is. Applying a cost-benefit framework can help.

Weighing the Costs and Benefits of Health Spending

As with any other government expenditure priority, it can be helpful to apply a cost-benefit analysis to health spending, even if only in abstract terms. Box 5.1 has further details. As discussed in chapter 2,

The Costs and Benefits of Health Spending

There are two types of social cost and two benefits associated with government health expenditures, as identified in public finance and health economics. The first cost is that of raising revenues to pay for the program (that is, the marginal cost of public funds), and the second is the moral hazard cost of excess health care utilization. On the benefit side, there are the value attached to improved health outcomes enabled by the spending program that would otherwise have been forgone for financial or behavioral reasons and the value of protection against financial risk caused by unpredictable out-of-pocket spending (depending on how "risk-averse" a person is and on the variability of health spending). These costs and benefits are shown in table B5.1.1. As long as the total social benefit exceeds the total social cost, health spending is on average "worth it." Additional spending is worth it if the same holds true on the margin. Otherwise, the spending may be justified on some other grounds, such as equity motives.

In practice, this calculation is difficult to carry out, as all four items are hard to measure. Some estimates have been made for the U.S. Medicare program in the years following its launch in 1965, suggesting that nearly half the social costs were recouped through the benefit of financial protection, although the health benefits were uncertain (Finkelstein and McKnight 2008). As discussed in chapter 2, the value of better health (measured as the willingness to pay for it) is very high, and rates of return for specific conditions well over 100 percent are not uncommon (table 2.1). As a result, health spending that is translated into a meaningful impact on outcomes will tend to have a favorable benefit-to-cost ratio. But if spending has no impact on health, or if it affords minimal financial protection, then the dual burden of the revenue raising and moral hazard will tend to dominate the equation, and the result may be significant waste. Overall, the evidence from richer countries is that while health spending has been worth it on average (that is, benefits have exceeded costs), there is also enormous waste on the margin (Cutler 2003).

TABLE B5.1.1

The Social Costs and Benefits of Government Health Spending

Costs	Benefits
Marginal cost of public funds	Value of better health
Moral hazard	Value of financial risk protection

Source: World Bank staff.

the cost-benefit calculus can be very favorable in health due to its high value, even in the presence of significant waste. The cost-benefit framework can also help put some of the foregoing discussion into context. The growth of health spending per se is not a cause for concern as long as the benefits exceed the costs. The efficiency agenda is about ensuring that this is indeed the case. More generally, the framework puts the focus on the ultimate objective of improving welfare.

The differences between growth of health spending and its efficiency, fiscal sustainability, and welfare implications as highlighted here suggest that it is important to be clear about what specific aspect of this agenda is being addressed. Table 5.1 provides a "Q&A" of commonly discussed issues, based on a similar exposition applied to the United States (Aaron and Ginsburg 2009). In the remainder of this chapter, we focus on how to cut back on spending without harming outcomes.

TABLE 5.1

Health Spending in ECA: Different Answers to Different Questions

Question	Answer
Does ECA spend more on health than the EU-15?	No. Government health budgets as a share of GDP are on average 4.3% in ECA, 8.0% in the EU-15.
Are health budgets rising faster in ECA than in the EU-15?	No. Health budgets in the EU-15 have risen faster on average as a percentage of GDP than almost all ECA countries.
Does ECA spend more on health than East Asia or Latin America?	Yes. It is also somewhat richer on average and much older than those regions (except for Central Asia).
Are health budgets rising faster in ECA than in East Asia or Latin America?	No. From 1997 to 2010, average annual growth as a percentage of GDP was higher in both East Asia and Latin America.
Are health systems in ECA wasteful?	Yes. All health systems worldwide would appear to have significant waste, perhaps 20 to 40 percent (WHO 2010).
Are health systems in ECA (relatively) more wasteful than those in the EU-15?	Unknown. In some respects, such as reliance on hospitals, almost certainly. In other areas, such as overuse of high-cost, low-value interventions, probably less wasteful.
Are medical care prices higher in ECA?	It depends. Salaries relative to national wages are generally lower in ECA than in the EU-15. Drug prices vary widely.
Do populations in ECA use more health care services than those in the EU-15?	Yes, on average. Outpatient visits per capita are slightly higher in ECA; acute-care hospital discharges per capita are higher. But there is significant country variation.
Do health systems in ECA provide less high-value, low-cost care than those in the EU-15?	Yes. Many cost-effective interventions, especially for prevention and management of risk factors, are underprovided in ECA.
Do ECA countries spend too much on health?	Unknown. Significant waste coexists with significant underprovision. Rates of return on health spending are potentially much higher than alternative public or private uses of these resources.
Are ECA health budgets fiscally sustainable?	It depends on other sectoral spending and tax policies.
Would higher health spending be a bad thing?	It depends. If the benefits of additional spending exceed the costs, no. If they do not, then yes.
Would cutting (growth of) health care spending in ECA raise welfare?	If one could target cuts to wasteful spending, yes; if not, no.

Source: World Bank staff.
Note: ECA = Europe and Central Asia; GDP = gross domestic product.

Hospitals and Pharmaceuticals Are the Main Sources of Waste

Inefficiency in health spending can come in many different forms. The WHO's World Health Report 2010 identified a "top 10" list of major sources of inefficiency in health systems around the world, reproduced in table 5.2. Many if not all are very relevant to ECA. In this section, we begin with a focus on hospitals and pharmaceuticals, both of which figure prominently on the list. Some of the other topics—such as quality of care—were discussed in previous chapters. The next section also touches on some of these causes of inefficiency.

The legacy of excess hospital infrastructure inherited from the pre-transition era is probably the best-known and most commonly analyzed efficiency problem in ECA's health systems. In fact, there is some variation across the region in the severity of the problem, both then and now. Historically, the western Balkans and Turkey did not overbuild to the same extent as Central and Eastern Europe and especially the Soviet Union. Since 1990, much progress has been made in rationalizing hospital capacity, and nowadays the problem remains acute mainly in the former Soviet republics (figure 5.2a). The EU-15 average also masks significant cross-country variation, and thus ECA can do better than that benchmark.

There are several dimensions to the problem of hospital waste. First, having too many hospitals (and often too many buildings *per* hospital) leads to high utility bills. In some countries, electricity and heating costs have accounted for as much as 20 percent or more of

TABLE 5.2

Ten Major Sources of Inefficiency in Health Systems Worldwide

Number	Cause
1	Underuse of generics and higher-than-necessary prices for medicines
2	Use of substandard and counterfeit medicines
3	Inappropriate and ineffective use of medicines
4	Overuse or supply of equipment, investigations, and procedures
5	Inappropriate or costly staff mix, unmotivated health workers
6	Inappropriate hospital admissions and length of stay
7	Inappropriate hospital size (low use of infrastructure)
8	Medical errors and suboptimal quality of care
9	Waste, corruption, and fraud
10	Inefficient mix of health interventions (for example, between prevention and treatment, high-value and low-value)

Source: WHO 2010.

FIGURE 5.2

A Lingering Challenge of Hospital Waste

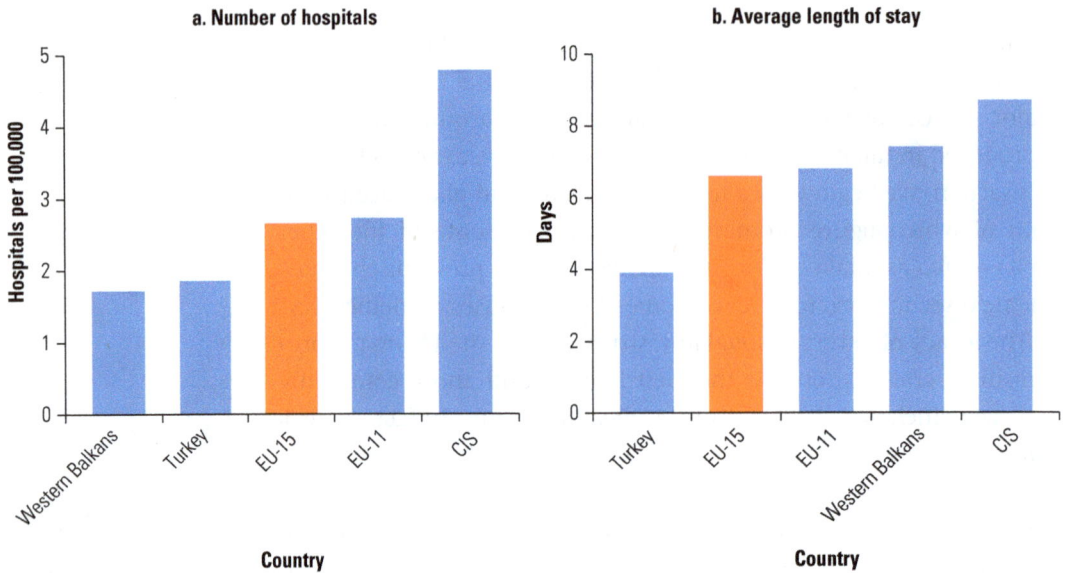

a. Number of hospitals

y-axis: Hospitals per 100,000 (0, 1, 2, 3, 4, 5)
x-axis (Country): Western Balkans, Turkey, EU-15, EU-11, CIS

b. Average length of stay

y-axis: Days (0, 2, 4, 6, 8, 10)
x-axis (Country): Turkey, EU-15, EU-11, Western Balkans, CIS

Source: WHO 2012b.
Note: Figure shows unweighted country averages. CIS = Commonwealth of Independent States.

total health spending (Haazen and Hayer 2010). Second, there is a tendency to justify excess hospital capacity by keeping patients admitted longer than necessary, as indicated by a higher average length of stay (figure 5.2b). This practice is both wasteful (absorbing other recurrent costs) and potentially harmful, since it needlessly exposes patients to hospital infections. Third, and related, people are admitted to hospital for the wrong reasons. For example, fewer than 1 per 1,000 adults in countries in the Organisation for Economic Co-operation and Development (OECD) is hospitalized due to hypertension, a condition that should be addressed through primary care; in all six countries in the former Soviet Union surveyed by the World Bank, more than 1 out of every 100 adults were hospitalized due to high blood pressure in the past year (OECD 2009b). Similarly, hospitals in ECA often serve as de facto long-term care facilities for the elderly, a role that should be shifted to social outreach to the extent possible. Fourth and finally, spreading service provision across a large number of facilities means less scope for specialization by providers, which evidence suggests will come at the expense of quality and thus value for money.

The downsizing of hospital networks is often achieved through a combination of decree and incentives. Hospital "master plans" have been applied in many countries and can help identify an optimal infrastructure mix with regard to coverage and cost, thereby guiding the consolidation process. The result may be both fewer hospitals and a better balance between multi- and single-profile facilities. These plans may also be applied to lower levels of care.

A widely cited success story with regard to hospital rationalization in ECA has been Estonia. In line with a hospital master plan, the total number of acute-care hospitals fell from over 100 to fewer than 40 between 1992 and 2002, and the average length of stay fell by about half over the same period. It also undertook reforms to change hospital status and created incentives for more efficient resource use (Haazen and Hayer 2010; Hawkins 2010).

In principle, reductions in hospital capacity can also be achieved through payment reforms such as selective contracting and a transition from input- to output-based payment schemes. For example, in recent years, Bulgaria has experienced a rapid increase in the number of hospitals in part because the national health insurance fund was obliged to contract with all newcomers, even if they were providing only the most lucrative services. Selective contracting could help in this respect but has faced resistance.

The promotion of service delivery innovations, such as one-day surgeries, can also complement efforts to save on hospital costs. Public-private partnerships may be a further option for improving hospital efficiency, especially if they serve to bring in stronger management expertise. It should be noted, however, that resolving excess or antiquated infrastructure may not result in aggregate cost savings, as significant investments in new or renovated facilities and equipment may also be required. But the result should be more efficient.

More often than not, however, the major obstacle to hospital rationalization has been political and not technical. Medical elites are often well connected and influential. Master plans are seen as suggestive only and thus subject to heavy lobbying. Moreover, the widespread reform of decentralizing hospital ownership in the 1990s often served to create vested interests among local leaders, for whom the hospital became a political asset that helped put the town on the map. Strong resistance to closure ensued. Thus, the hospital reform agenda is to a large extent about making difficult political decisions.

An even more widespread cause of inefficient health spending in ECA is the pharmaceutical sector. We saw in chapter 4 that drugs account for a major share of out-of-pocket spending, in part because of high prices that arise from a lack of purchasing power when drugs are not covered in benefit packages. But excess drug spending is not limited to OOP expenditures. Governments across the region are struggling to contain the pressure drugs exert on their own budgets.

A larger share of total health spending is being allocated to drugs in ECA than in the EU-15 (figure 5.3).

One challenge is high prices. In many countries, there is scope for procurement reform and more "smart purchasing" of drugs, including a preference for generic instead of brand-name drugs, external reference pricing, the regulation of margins, claw-backs, price-volume contracts, and a systematic review of reimbursement policies, especially for high-cost drugs (Seiter 2010). Box 5.2 shows how some of these measures helped Croatia successfully control its drug budget in recent years.

FIGURE 5.3

Overdosing on Pharmaceutical Spending

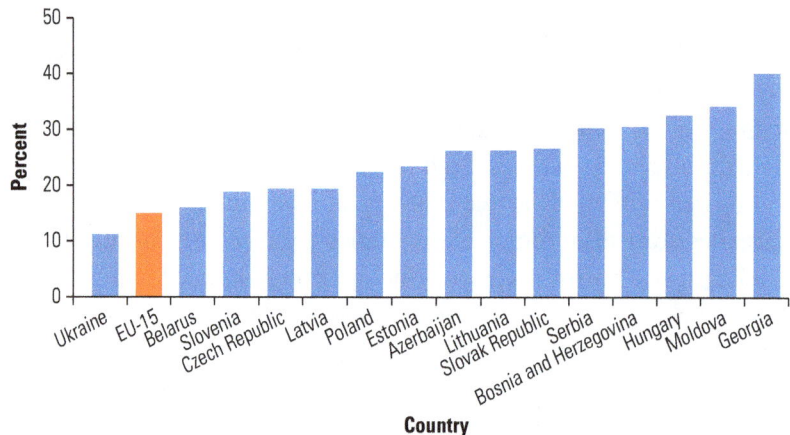

Source: WHO 2012b.
Note: Figure shows pharmaceutical spending as a percentage of total health spending in selected countries in Europe and Central Asia and in the EU-15, 2009.

BOX 5.2

Successful Cost Containment of Pharmaceuticals in Croatia

After several years of growing cost pressures, during 2009–10 Croatia substantially reformed its regulations related to the pricing and reimbursement of medicines with the aim of achieving better value for money. Reforms included greater transparency in decision making; a stronger role for evidence-based medicine and health economic criteria; and so-called rebate, payback, and cross-product agreements in contracting with pharmaceutical companies, among other measures. As a result of these steps, expenditure on prescription medicines fell by 13 percent between 2009 and 2010, while spending on expensive hospital medicines decreased by 29 percent (Voncina and Strizrep 2010).

Another challenge is overconsumption. The rational use of medicines is a responsibility of doctors and patients alike. A recent study in Kazakhstan found that over 90 percent of the population self-medicates. Prescription guidelines and monitoring can help. When primary care is weak, these mechanisms are also weakened. In some cases, the challenge is compounded by direct payment of physicians by pharmaceutical companies in exchange for favorable prescription patterns. But some of the responsibility is on patients as well, who may be asked to pay higher copayments for brand-name drugs and should be targeted with information to help overcome potential bias against drugs with a certain country of origin.

No Silver Bullets

Having seen the potential for cutting waste in hospitals and pharmaceuticals, we should also note that there are some commonly proposed "cures" for health inefficiency for which the evidence is not without important caveats. In principle, provider payment reforms such as the adoption of diagnosis-related groups can improve efficiency, but in practice, the evidence is not so clear (Street et al. 2011). More cost sharing, prevention programs, and competition are also frequently proposed as policy instruments for improving efficiency. But in each case, the evidence is mixed. Similarly, certain broad health system models are sometimes viewed as inherently more efficient, but a recent analysis has cast doubt on any such clear conclusions (OECD 2010). These are briefly summarized in table 5.3.

TABLE 5.3

No Easy Answers for the Efficiency Agenda

Potential efficiency-enhancing policy	Possible side effects
More cost sharing	Patients may cut back on preventive care and end up with higher rates of hospitalization; see box 4.1 for evidence. Ultimately likely to vary by service.
More prevention	Very important for improving health, but may not decrease (lifetime) costs; for example, smokers tend to have lower lifetime medical costs than nonsmokers because they live much shorter lives (Sloan et al. 2004). Overall, prevention may be no cheaper than treatment (Cohen, Neumann, and Weinstein 2008).
More insurer competition	May induce innovation and cut back on wasteful care, but could also result in higher systemwide administrative costs, higher prices due to loss of monopsony power, and cutbacks of "necessary care" such as prevention.
More provider competition	May improve incentives to cut costs, but this may be done by skimping on quality of care. Empirical evidence is ambiguous (Gaynor and Town 2012).
Type of health system in country X	There is more variation in efficiency within broad health system types than across them (OECD 2010).

Source: World Bank staff.

Together they suggest that there are few easy answers to be applied to the efficiency agenda. In the next section, we turn to a more nuanced approach that may hold more promise.

Cutting the Fat but Not the Muscle

One of the biggest challenges posed by the efficiency agenda is that while health systems often have a large amount of waste, at the same time they provide some very high value care, and it can be difficult to cut one without cutting the other. For example, some services may be overprovided while others are underprovided. A procedure that is life saving for one patient may be useless for another. How can a ministry of finance or health distinguish between them? It is in this sense that an agenda of cost containment may or may not improve welfare when a "macro" policy is applied across the board. In this section, we give some examples and possible approaches for addressing the "micro" challenge.

While an important target for efforts to improve the efficiency of the health system should be to cut back on wasteful or unnecessary care, some caution is warranted when doing so. Figure 5.4 gives

FIGURE 5.4

Overprovision and Underprovision Coexist in All Health Systems

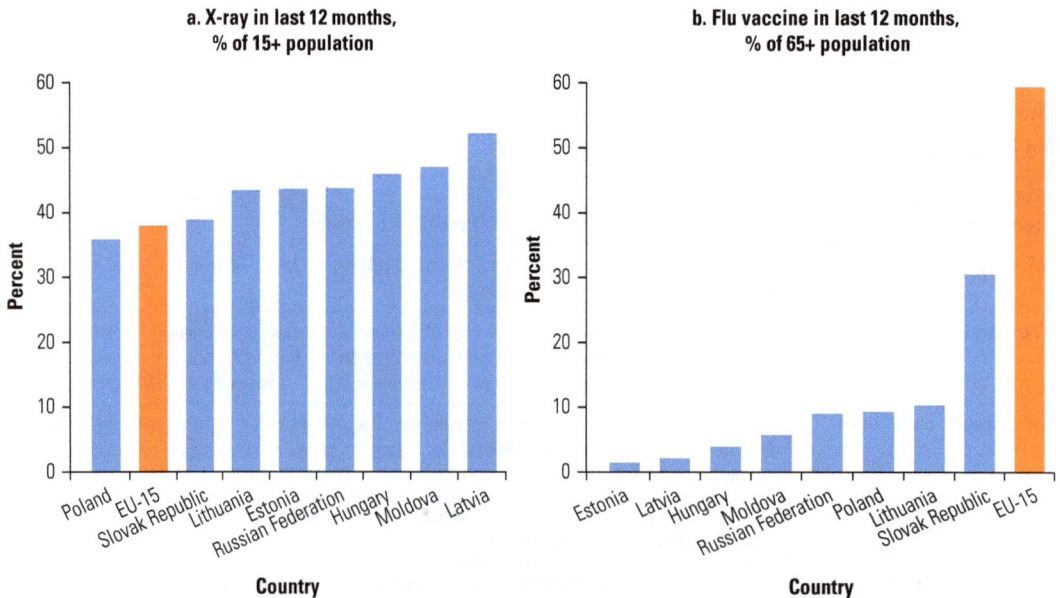

Sources: European Commission 2007; OECD 2011; Venice II Consortium 2011; World Bank 2012.
Note: Figure shows provision of X-rays and flu vaccine in selected countries in Europe and Central Asia and in the EU-15.

two examples. Figure 5.4a shows that several ECA countries perform X-rays significantly more often than is the case in Western Europe. While we cannot know for certain that some country or region is doing just the "right" number, it is likely that because in the past many ECA countries trained a large number of X-ray technicians and installed the equipment, there is a tendency to make use of these resources more than is necessary. Not only is this wasteful, but it could also be harmful.

Figure 5.4b provides a counterexample using the same countries. Influenza is a common ailment that in some cases may lead to serious complications, especially among the elderly. As a result, it is widely recommended that those with chronic conditions and older popula-tions receive a flu vaccine annually. Yet very few elderly people in ECA receive a seasonal flu vaccine compared to those in the EU-15. This is a low-cost (and potentially cost-saving) service that should be provided more often.

There are many more examples like these, some of which were seen in chapter 3. To be successful, the efficiency agenda must find a way to cut back on services like X-rays while expanding interventions like flu vaccines. Across-the-board reforms to provider payment methods or cost-sharing policies may be too blunt to accomplish this task. Adapting these instruments for different types of services—such as value-based cost sharing noted in box 4.1—offers more promise.

More generally, it is possible to identify broad classes of health care services with the aim of tailoring the efficiency agenda accord-ingly. Table 5.4 distinguishes three types based on a recent formulation (Chandra and Skinner 2012). The first category is highly cost-effective care that is useful for nearly everyone in the relevant population (in the examples given in the table, those with cardiovascular disease or HIV) and is thus unlikely to result in

TABLE 5.4

Different Technologies Imply Different Policy Agendas for Improving Efficiency

Service type	Examples	Possible policy response
Highly cost-effective interventions	Cheap cardiovascular disease drugs; anti-retrovirals	Not a major spending (efficiency) concern
Highly cost-effective interventions for some patients, not for others	Stents; CT scans; MRIs	Monitor volumes; measure outcomes (by provider)
Interventions with low or uncertain cost-effectiveness	New cancer drugs; some knee and back surgeries	Comparative effectiveness research

Source: World Bank staff.
Note: CT = computed tomography; MRI = magnetic resonance imaging.

overspending. The second type includes services that are very cost effective for some patients but not for others. Many diagnostic services and some treatments would fall in this group. The third category includes high-cost services whose clinical effectiveness is unknown. This last group calls for careful design of benefit packages and potentially the establishment of institutions to undertake comparative effectiveness research (of which a particularly well-known example is the United Kingdom's National Institute for Health and Clinical Excellence).

The second category—those with heterogeneous benefits—poses a particularly challenging case for improving efficiency. Take the example of stents, or small mesh tubes that help treat coronary artery blockages in those with heart disease. Some patients benefit enormously from this technology, and indeed stents are credited with making an important contribution to the decline of cardiovascular disease mortality in recent years. But many people with heart problems do not need stents—either because their condition is not serious enough or because it is too advanced and thus more aggressive procedures are required. To add another layer of complexity, stents may or may not be drug eluting, which are helpful in some but not all cases and are certainly more expensive. Improving efficiency requires a systemwide mechanism to help figure out who will benefit from stents and who will not.

There is an important role for strengthening information flows and analytical capacity to address this dimension of the efficiency agenda. Monitoring the volume of services and outcomes at the provider level can shed light on which corners of the health system are generating the most waste. For example, figure 5.5 shows the regional variation in hospitalizations for pneumonia in Bulgaria. This is a condition that should generally be handled either at primary care or on an ambulatory basis at hospital. Most regions are well above the OECD average, indicating a nationwide problem, but significant gains could be made just by targeting the worst offenders (where discharges are nearly 10 times the OECD rate).

In many cases, unnecessary care may not reflect deliberate rent seeking by providers but instead arises because in the absence of clear evidence—there is a substantial "gray area" in the practice of medicine—clinical decision making may be driven by individual or community behavioral norms ("that's how it's always done"). Information feedback can help change this reality. This issue is discussed further in chapter 6.

FIGURE 5.5

Identifying and Addressing Outliers Can Help Promote Efficiency Gains

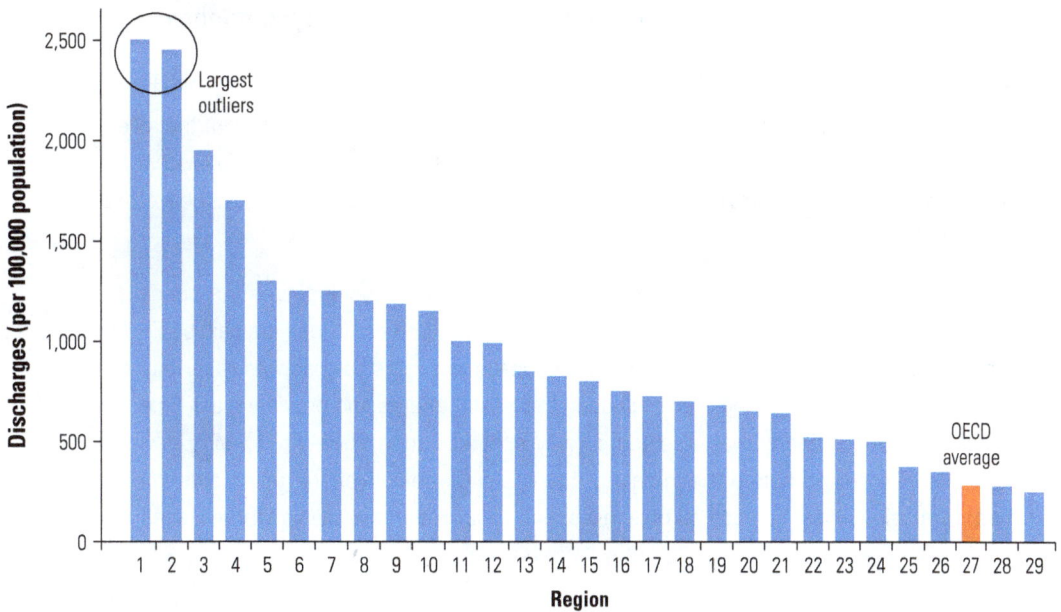

Source: World Bank data.
Note: Figure shows hospital discharges for pneumonia in Bulgaria, by region. OECD = Organisation for Economic Co-operation and Development.

Indeed, approaching the efficiency agenda from a "micro" angle applies equally to individual providers as well as to services. The organizations that pay for services should keep track of patterns such as which doctors refer the most patients to higher levels of care or which doctors prescribe the most drugs or which hospitals have the highest readmission rates or mortality rates for specific types of care. There may be good reasons why some facilities are outliers—for example, the best hospitals may get the most difficult cases. But sometimes there is not a good reason. More active purchasing within an existing system may yield more benefits in some circumstances than changing the purchasing system altogether.

In sum, an important part of the efficiency agenda is not about pursuing major systemic reforms. Instead, understanding cross-country data on service provision and within-country variation in outputs and outcomes by provider and service type can point the way toward significant efficiency gains. In many instances, the right instrument for the cost-cutting agenda will be a scalpel and not a sword. Box 5.3 provides an example of selective cutbacks in the context of an economic crisis, based on the Estonian experience.

Making Cutbacks during an Economic Crisis: The Estonian Experience

The global financial crisis of 2008–09 struck Estonia particularly hard, with real GDP shrinking by almost 15 percent in 2009. The extent of the required fiscal consolidation meant that every sector had to make a contribution to macroeconomic recovery. The task for the Ministry of Health and Estonian Health Insurance Fund (EHIF) was to find budget cuts that would have the least harmful side effects.

Among the cost-cutting initiatives were higher limits on waiting times, a cancellation of dental benefits for adults, reduced sick leave benefits for workers (these are paid by EHIF) especially for short-duration illnesses, and higher copayment rates for patients receiving inpatient nursing care. To ensure some burden sharing between patients and providers, a 3–5 percent cut in reimbursement prices was also temporarily applied during 2010–11. Drawing down EHIF's reserves also helped soften the impact of the crisis. By selectively targeting cuts, the authorities were able to balance sectoral objectives with fiscal imperatives (Ministry of Health 2012).

References

Aaron, H., and P. Ginsburg. 2009. "Is Health Spending Excessive? If So, What Can We Do about It?" *Health Affairs* 28 (5): 1260–75.

Chandra, A., and J. Skinner. 2012. "Technology Growth and Expenditure Growth in Health Care." *Journal of Economic Literature* 50 (3): 645–80.

Chernew, M., and J. Newhouse. 2012. "Health Care Spending Growth." In *Handbook of Health Economics*, vol. 2, edited by Mark V. Pauly, Thomas G. McGuire, and Pedro P. Barros, 1–43. Oxford: Elsevier Science BV.

Cohen, J. T., P. J. Neumann, and M. C. Weinstein. 2008. "Does Preventive Care Save Money?" *New England Journal of Medicine* 358: 661–63.

Cutler, D. M. 2003. "A Framework for Evaluating Medical Care Systems." In *A Disease-Based Comparison of Health Systems: What Is Best and at What Cost?* OECD, 121–30. OECD: Paris.

European Commission. 2007. *Eurobarometer* 66.2, October–November 2006. TNS Opinion & Social, Brussels. GESIS Data Archive ZA4527, dataset version 1.0.

———. 2010. "Joint Report on Health Systems." European Economy Occasional Paper 74, European Commission, Brussels.

Finkelstein, A., and R. McKnight. 2008. "What Did Medicare Do? The Initial Impact of Medicare on Mortality and Out of Pocket Medical Spending." *Journal of Public Economics* 92: 1644–69.

Gaynor, M., and R. Town. 2012. "Competition in Health Care Markets." In *Handbook of Health Economics*, vol. 2, edited by Mark V. Pauly, Thomas G. McGuire, and Pedro P. Barros, 499–637. Oxford: Elsevier Science BV.

Haazen, D. S., and A. S. Hayer. 2010. "Financing Capital Costs and Reducing the Fixed Costs of Health Systems." In *Implementing Health Financing Reform: Lessons from Countries in Transition,* edited by J. Kutzin, C. Cashin, and M. Jakab, 221–46. Copenhagen: WHO Euro Observatory.

Hall, R. E., and C. I. Jones. 2007. "The Value of Life and the Rise in Health Spending." *Quarterly Journal of Economics* 122 (1): 39–72.

Hawkins, L. 2010. "Optimization of Hospital Capacity: Lessons from the Estonian Experience." Draft. World Bank, Washington, DC.

Hollingsworth, B. 2008. "The Measurement of Efficiency and Productivity of Health Care Delivery." *Health Economics* 17: 1107–28.

IMF (International Monetary Fund). 2012. *The Economics of Public Health Care Reform in Advanced and Emerging Economies.* Washington, DC: International Monetary Fund.

Ministry of Health, Estonia. 2012. "Sustainability of Health Financing in Estonia." Presentation at OECD Senior Budget Officials Meeting, June 28–29, Tallinn.

Newhouse, J. P. 1994. "Frontier Estimation: How Useful A Tool for Health Economics?" *Journal of Health Economics* 13: 317–22.

OECD (Organisation for Economic Co-operation and Development). 2009a. *Achieving Better Value for Money in Health Care.* Paris: Organisation for Economic Co-operation and Development.

———. 2009b. *Health at a Glance.* Paris: Organisation for Economic Co-operation and Development.

———. 2010. *Health Care Systems: Efficiency and Institutions.* Paris: Organisation for Economic Co-operation and Development.

———. 2011. *OECD Health at a Glance 2011: OECD Indicators.* Paris: Organisation for Economic Co-operation and Development.

Seiter, A. 2010. *A Practical Approach to Pharmaceutical Policy.* Washington, DC: World Bank.

Sloan, F., J. Ostermann, G. Picone, C. Conover, and D. H. Taylor. 2004. *The Price of Smoking.* Cambridge, MA: MIT Press.

Street, A., J. O'Reilly, P. Ward, and A. Mason. 2011. "DRG-Based Hospital Payment and Efficiency: Theory, Evidence, and Challenges." In *Diagnosis-Related Groups in Europe,* edited by R. Busse, A. Geissler, W. Quentin, and M. Wiley. 93–114. Brussels: WHO European Observatory.

Venice II Consortium. 2011. *Seasonal Influenza Vaccination Survey in EU/EEA.* http://venice.cineca.org/Final_Seasonal_Influenza_Vaccination_Survey_2010.pdf.

Voncina, L., and T. Strizrep. 2010. "Croatia: 2009/2010 Pharmaceutical Pricing and Reimbursement Reform." *Eurohealth* 16 (4): 20–22.

WHO (World Health Organization). 2010. *World Health Report—Health Systems Financing: The Path to Universal Coverage.* Geneva: World Health Organization.

———. 2012a. National Health Accounts (database), World Health Organization, Geneva, http://www.who.int/nha/expenditure_database/en.

————. 2012b. Health for All (database), World Health Organization, Geneva, http://www.euro.who.int/en/what-we-do/data-and-evidence/databases/ european-health-for-all-database-hfa-db2.

World Bank. 2007. "Health Care Spending in the New EU Member States: Controlling Costs and Improving Quality." Working Paper 113, World Bank, Washington, DC.

————. 2012. "Findings from a Household Survey on Health in 6 ECA Countries." Draft. World Bank, Washington, DC.

CHAPTER 6

Improving Institutions: Ingredients, Not Recipes

Key Messages

- Major health reform themes in ECA over the past 20 years have included hospital downsizing, the establishment of family medicine for primary care, the introduction of new health financing arrangements, the decentralization of facility ownership, and the creation of new public health structures.

- Identifying ECA's unfinished institutional reform agenda is complicated by the fact that it is not immediately clear what a "developed" health system looks like. A systematic comparison of the institutional characteristics of health systems in ECA and OECD countries helps shed light on this question.

- With respect to health financing, nearly all OECD countries have converged toward high levels of population coverage, but their approaches to revenue raising and risk pooling differ substantially. The health financing policy agenda for ECA is thus mainly to expand coverage, with more than a single institutional approach available for doing so.

- Patterns of facility ownership and provider payment in ECA are more similar to the OECD in the hospital sector than in primary care, where a significant agenda remains for achieving institutional convergence with more advanced health systems.

- In view of the diversity of OECD health systems, there are no simple, clear recipes for health reform that can be distilled from their experience, only a few key ingredients.

- The first three ingredients of successful health systems that we identify here are all strongly tied to the concept of *accountability*. These are: (1) some element of activity-based payment; (2) provider autonomy; and (3) information for decision making.

- Two additional ingredients for health reform are also identified. One is a health financing system that achieves adequate risk pooling without extensive fragmentation, and the other is strong leadership commitment.

- Part of ECA's health sector challenge is to achieve a greater degree of institutional convergence by incorporating these key ingredients into its health system reforms.

The three previous chapters have examined the policy agenda related to three major objectives of all health systems: to improve health outcomes, financial protection, and the efficiency of spending. But these issues have been explored independently, without paying much attention to the overall institutional design of the health system. As noted at the outset, the aim has been to focus on results, which implies starting with the specific objective in mind and then proceeding to "work backward" to identify the appropriate policy instruments. But ultimately this process brings us to the question of how to strengthen the underlying institutions that affect all three of the major objectives already discussed.

This chapter assesses the extent to which the slow convergence of key outcomes between Europe and Central Asia (ECA) and its comparators as highlighted earlier is due to a lack of institutional convergence. But this task poses a challenge, since it is not immediately obvious what a "developed" health system looks like. As a result, it is more difficult to benchmark ECA's health systems against the *institutions* of advanced countries than, for example, against the health *outcomes* of those countries. Thus, a key message of the chapter is that because there is considerable diversity among successful health systems in advanced countries, there is no simple "recipe" for reform, only a list of "ingredients" that appear common to most if not all successful health systems. It is on this basis that an agenda for improving the institutions governing ECA's health systems can be identified.

The chapter begins with a brief review of the broad themes of health reform in ECA since transition. It then compares the institutional characteristics of the region's health systems with those in countries of the Organisation for Economic Co-operation and Development (OECD) and draws on this comparison to help identify the outlines of a reform agenda going forward. The topics addressed range from how the health sector is financed (revenue generation, pooling, and purchasing); how service delivery is organized (public-private mix, patient pathways); and regulatory arrangements (affecting hospital management, information flows, and so forth). These issues are of course the subject of a vast literature, both in ECA and worldwide. Here we can take only a broad-brush approach—the finer details of each topic are explored more thoroughly in those other sources.

A Brief History of Health Reform in ECA since the Transition

The story of health reform in ECA over the past 20 years necessarily begins with the historical legacy of the pretransition health systems. The so-called Semashko system that prevailed in the Soviet republics was characterized by central planning and administration, government-owned facilities with an overemphasis on hospital care, and publicly employed staff who were mostly specialists. In principle, there was free universal coverage with funding from general government revenue sources, although health systems did not always live up to this promise. Primary care was not emphasized, and public health was narrowly focused on infectious diseases. The system was inefficient, and evidence-based medicine was only weakly applied. The countries of Central and Eastern Europe had health systems broadly similar to the Soviet model in most respects. The Yugoslav republics also had many of these same features but with some important differences, including an employer-based health insurance model, greater emphasis on primary care, and, for a while, higher funding levels (Davis 2010).

Much of the posttransition reform agenda has involved unwinding or overcoming this legacy. As we shall see later in this chapter, this agenda remains unfinished. Much has been written about the reform experience (World Bank 2000; Figueras et al. 2004; Borowitz and Atun 2006; Rechel and McKee 2009; Kutzin, Cashin, and Jakab 2010). This section only briefly touches on some of the major themes.

Perhaps the most widespread reform task undertaken by ECA health systems since transition has been to downsize the hospital sector to rationalize service provision and improve system efficiency. As of 1990, most of the erstwhile Soviet republics had nearly 1,000 hospital beds per 100,000 population, or nearly three times the standard level in Western Europe. In Central and Eastern Europe, it was almost twice as high. During the past two decades, the number of hospital beds has been cut by over 50 percent in Central Asia and the south Caucasus, where the posttransition fiscal collapse was most severe, and by about a third in Belarus, Moldova, Ukraine, and the new EU member states. There have also been significant declines in the number of hospitals. These optimization programs have typically involved reconfiguring and relocating services, often with reference to a master plan. Nevertheless, more needs to be done on this front in many ECA countries.

A related priority has been the establishment of a family medicine model for primary care. Neglected in the previous system but motivated by the Western European experience, primary care became a focal point of the reform agenda in many countries. Major activities included retraining and recertifying medical staff and introducing family medicine into medical curricula. Since family medicine was not previously an academic discipline or commonplace in the community, changing attitudes within the profession and among the population was a key challenge. A related task has been the reform of polyclinics, the outpatient centers staffed by narrow specialists that have proven difficult to change (Rechel and McKee 2008, 2009). Overall, the establishment of primary care has been a mixed success thus far, with significant variation in experience across countries (World Bank 2005).

In many countries of Central and Eastern Europe, these service delivery reforms were accompanied on the health financing side by the creation of social insurance schemes and the enforcement of a purchaser-provider split. In some cases, these health financing reforms entailed a return to social health insurance (SHI) systems that had existed earlier in the 20th century. More generally, a major consideration in the post-Communist era was to repeal the centralized authority of the state by creating an independent SHI agency with a steady funding flow and freeing provision from the constraints imposed by a sclerotic state. To a lesser extent, this pattern also unfolded in some post-Soviet states. This regionwide SHI "experiment" also ushered in new provider payment mechanisms, typically a shift from historical budgets to fee-for-service or approaches based on diagnosis-related groups (DRGs) (Wagstaff and Moreno-Serra 2009; Moreno-Serra and Wagstaff 2010).

A related theme has been the decentralization of hospital owner-ship from the ministries of health to municipalities in many coun-tries, again motivated partly by a desire to roll back the influence of central authorities and partly in the hope that local entities would be more responsive to population wishes. But this decentralization has arguably created as many problems as it has solved, as the hospitals became local political assets that SHI agencies had to contract with and could not shut down, thus hindering rationalization policies. Moreover, their municipal owners did not impose hard budget con-straints, as funding flows and bailouts still came from the center (Preker and Harding 2003).

A final reform area of note has been public health. Historically, the sanitary-epidemiological system was hierarchical and top heavy and had little interface with the population. In some countries, this real-ity has persisted, while in others, it has been replaced outright, while in still others, new and old structures operate side by side. Generally, these systems have been more successful at sustaining long-standing vaccination programs but less so at promoting health, especially as it applies to noncommunicable diseases. These systems have also strug-gled to deal with new challenges such as HIV/AIDS (Maier and Martin-Moreno 2011).

Finally, it bears mentioning that "health reform" is arguably a journey and not a destination, as nearly all advanced health systems have also been subject to ongoing health reform initiatives in recent decades. Major themes have included improving both access to and quality of care while maintaining fiscal sustainability (Docteur and Oxley 2003). Health reform in rich countries has followed a pattern whereby the main objectives of new initiatives have alternated between better access and equity on the one hand (for example, through coverage expansions or supply-side invest-ments) and efficiency on the other (spending controls and cost sharing, for example) and then back again, depending on fiscal imperatives and popular views of the day (Cutler 2002). It has been argued that, over time, OECD reforms have converged toward "mixed systems" that balance regulation and market mechanisms (Rothgang 2010).

Where Are We Now? A Comparison of ECA and OECD Health Systems

While the health sector has been an active area of reform over the past 20 years throughout ECA, a significant unfinished agenda remains. But to identify *what* remains to be done, we need some understanding of the destination. That knowledge is relatively clear with respect to outcomes—for example, we have seen how ECA compares to the EU-15 in life expectancy, the incidence of catastrophic health expenditures, and government health spending. But it is more difficult in the case of the institutional features of health systems. What does a "developed" health system look like? And how do ECA's health systems compare?

A systematic assessment of the institutional characteristics of ECA health systems was undertaken during 2011–12 to help answer these questions, using an abridged version of a questionnaire developed by the OECD and implemented in its member countries in 2009 (Paris, Devaux, and Wei 2010). The survey covered a broad range of topics related to health financing, service delivery, organization, and governance. Together, these yield a rich overview of health system characteristics in over 50 countries around the world, as the OECD includes non-European countries such as Australia, Canada, Japan, the Republic of Korea, Mexico, and New Zealand (the United States, which has many varied health systems rolled into one, did not participate).

The two major questions to be addressed through this exercise are as follows. First, to what extent have the institutional characteristics of the OECD's health systems converged? And second, where this convergence has occurred, to what extent have ECA health systems also evolved toward this common approach? This section summarizes the main results. Of necessity, it involves a bird's-eye view of health system characteristics: the reality of everyday implementation is more complex and nuanced. Nevertheless, it reveals an informative picture of how OECD and ECA systems compare.

To better organize the findings, we compare the OECD (excluding those countries that are also in ECA) with "ECA West," comprised of the new EU member states, the western Balkans, and Turkey (a group that includes several OECD members), and "ECA East," the non-Baltic countries of the former Soviet Union.

Health Financing: Convergence on Coverage Levels, Not Institutions

We begin with the institutional arrangements for health financing. Figure 6.1 shows how countries address two fundamental policy issues in this area. The first is whether health coverage is "automatic"—that is, based on residence or citizenship and funded through general taxes—or "compulsory" in the form of mandatory income-based contributions to a social health insurance scheme. Within the OECD, countries are nearly evenly split between the two models. In reality, many in the latter group have a hybrid system, with supplementary transfers from general tax revenues to cover those outside the formal SHI system. In the western part of ECA, the predominant model is mandatory contributions, as noted. In the eastern countries, automatic coverage is the norm, with only Moldova and the Russian Federation relying mainly on a contributory system. Georgia has neither model, as enrollment in its largest coverage program was voluntary as of 2012.

A second related dimension of health financing policy is whether coverage is achieved in the form of national (or local) health services or through an insurance pool with either a single or multiple

FIGURE 6.1

Significant Diversity of Health Financing Arrangements within the OECD and across ECA

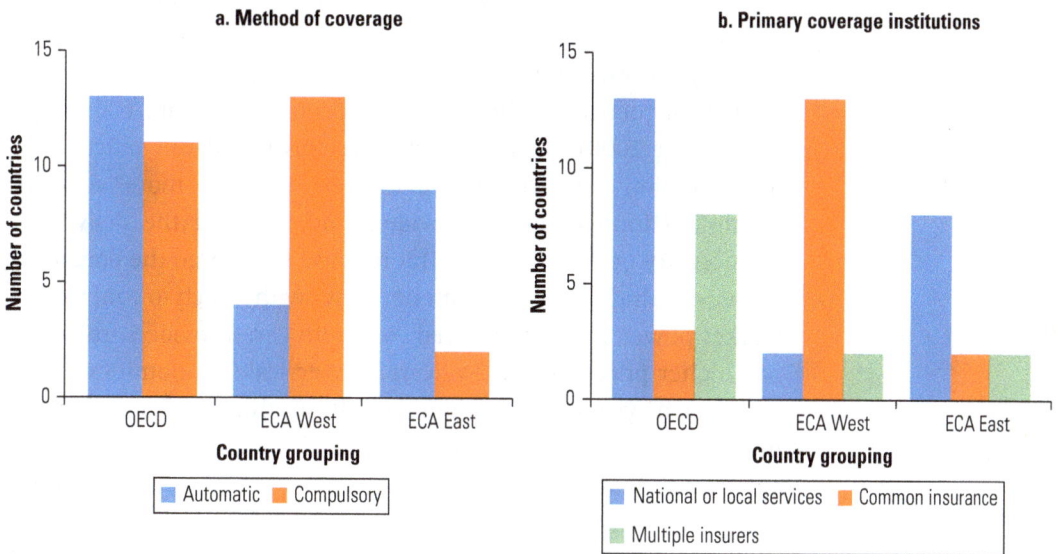

a. Method of coverage

b. Primary coverage institutions

Legend (a): ■ Automatic ■ Compulsory

Legend (b): ■ National or local services ■ Common insurance ■ Multiple insurers

Sources: Paris, Devaux, and Wei 2010; World Bank 2012.

Note: Figure shows the organization of health financing in ECA and the OECD. ECA = Europe and Central Asia; OECD = Organisation for Economic Co-operation and Development.

insurers. Again, there is significant variety among OECD countries, with the contributory systems further divided into three countries with a single insurance pool and eight relying on multiple insurers, of which five do not extend any choice of insurer to the patient, while three do allow choice. The western part of ECA relies mainly on common insurance pools, while national health services predominate farther east, but there are exceptions to the rule in both regions.

What does the evidence say about alternative health financing approaches? The relative merits of general tax or SHI-based financing of health care have been the subject of much debate (Wagstaff 2010). Evidence from Western Europe and Asia suggests that tax-financed systems are generally more progressive with regard to how revenues are raised, and they do a better job of ensuring universal coverage, whereas SHI systems often leave certain vulnerable groups such as informal workers and the poor uncovered. SHI systems may also have a negative impact on the labor market due to the distortions created by a payroll tax and higher administrative costs due to parallel structures. But it is also sometimes argued that they generate a larger, more reliable flow of funds to the health sector. However, there is less evidence on the comparative performance of tax and SHI-based systems with respect to actual health outcomes among those who are covered under the different approaches.

Similarly, much has been written about the pros and cons of opting for a single or for multiple purchasers. The competitive pressures of a multiple insurer model may offer the hope of greater efficiency, but this hope comes with several caveats. In an unregulated market, the tendency will be to compete on the consumer side by denying coverage to high-risk individuals, leading to market failure with consequences for financial protection and welfare (Cutler and Zeckhauser 2000). Most advanced systems forbid this practice. On the provision side, competing insurers may be more active in promoting innovation by providers and reducing the delivery of unnecessary or wasteful care. But because they forgo the bargaining power of a single purchaser (monopsony) with which to confront the market power typically enjoyed by health care providers, they may pay higher prices for medical care. Fewer scale economies can also mean such systems incur higher administrative costs, and the fragmentation of risk pools can result in greater inequalities in access and coverage. Greater consumer choice of insurance plans is another potential benefit, but the complexity of the product may be a barrier to making better decisions. In reality, most advanced systems with multiple insurers have extensive regulations that help mitigate these issues. Overall, empirical evidence does not give clear-cut answers on the relative efficiency of the different insurance models as currently applied (Gaynor and Town 2012; OECD 2010).

Against a background of inconclusive evidence on the relative merits of different approaches, perhaps the main conclusion to draw from an overview of health financing arrangements across the OECD is that while there is limited convergence on institutional structures, greater similarities exist in coverage. In most OECD countries and for most services (for example, hospital and primary care, lab tests, and drugs), benefit packages cover at least 75 percent of the cost (figure 6.2a). This coverage is also generally the case in the western part of ECA, with the exception of drugs. In eastern ECA, there are sizable gaps in coverage across all services.

The convergence in OECD coverage is also reflected in the levels of government health spending and financial protection as indicated by reliance on out-of-pocket (OOP) spending. Figure 6.2a shows that most OECD countries are clustered in a range between 7 and 9 percent of gross domestic product (GDP) spent on health, with OOP spending accounting for less than 20 percent of total health expenditure. Outliers are mostly those with somewhat lower income—Greece, the Republic of Korea, and Mexico. Indeed, a detailed study of OECD data between 1970 and 2005 found convergence in public health spending both per capita and as a share of total health spending (Leiter and

FIGURE 6.2

OECD Has Converged toward High Coverage Levels but ECA Has Not

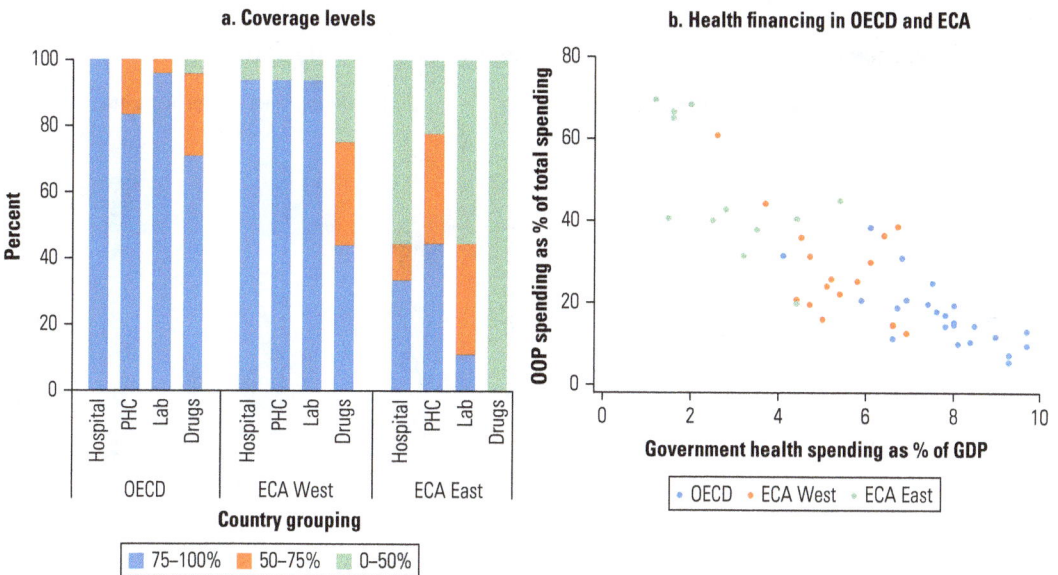

a. Coverage levels

b. Health financing in OECD and ECA

Sources: Paris, Devaux, and Wei 2010; World Bank 2012; WHO 2012.
Note: ECA = Europe and Central Asia; GDP = gross domestic product; OECD = Organisation for Economic Co-operation and Development; OOP = out of pocket; PHC = primary health care.

Theurl 2010). The countries with lower initial spending levels experienced higher growth and vice versa. This convergence has unfolded even while institutional approaches differ widely.

What does such convergence mean for ECA? It should be clear that a variety of health financing structures is consistent with good overall outcomes, with regard both to health and to financial protection. For equity purposes, it is important that risk-pooling arrangements should not be too fragmented. The equity concerns with SHI-based systems can be mitigated through transfers from general taxes. Perhaps the major argument against a payroll-tax-based health financing system is the (nonhealth) issue of the distortion imposed on labor markets. It is also clear that no advanced health system relies heavily on private voluntary health insurance. Otherwise, the health financing agenda should arguably focus on improving coverage and outcomes irrespective of the prevailing institutional arrangements, which in any event are usually the outcome of a long historical legacy and thus are unlikely to be easily undone.

Ownership and Provider Payment: More Differences between ECA and OECD in Primary Care

We next turn to the question of facility ownership. For the provision of primary care, 17 out of 24 OECD countries rely on private providers (figure 6.3). These may be either private solo or group

FIGURE 6.3

Greater Differences between ECA and OECD in Ownership of Primary Care than Hospitals

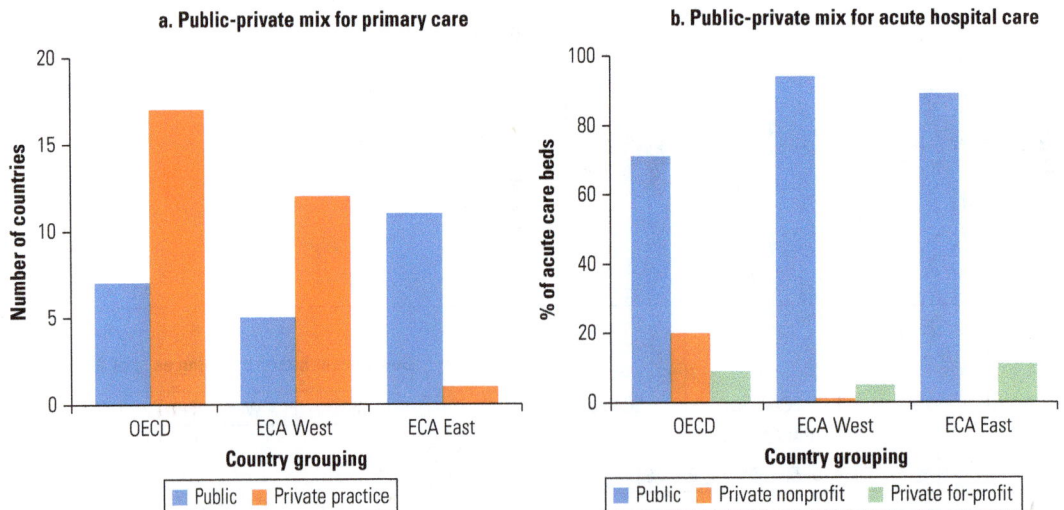

a. Public-private mix for primary care

b. Public-private mix for acute hospital care

Sources: Paris, Devaux, and Wei 2010; World Bank 2012.
Note: Figure shows the ownership of facilities. ECA = Europe and Central Asia; OECD = Organisation for Economic Co-operation and Development.

practices, with the former being more common. Seven of the 17 relying on private providers cover their populations through national health services as described above: Australia, Canada, Denmark, Ireland, New Zealand, Norway, and the United Kingdom. These correspond to what has been called the public contracting model, with public finance and private provision, a hybrid between the public integrated model and private insurance and provision model (Docteur and Oxley 2003). Public provision of primary care is found in seven OECD countries, mostly in the Mediterranean or Scandinavian regions: Finland, Iceland, Italy, Mexico, Portugal, Spain, and Sweden. (Here and below we rely on national data for Spain and Sweden, while noting that there are differences across regions within these countries with respect to some health system characteristics.) But Finland, Mexico, and Sweden have a secondary reliance on private practice. Thus, full reliance on public primary care is increasingly rare.

A similar public-private mix for primary care is found in the western part of the ECA region, with public centers more common in the former Yugoslavia (except Croatia and the former Yugoslav Republic of Macedonia) and private primary care the norm in new EU member states. In the eastern part of ECA, publicly provided primary care is the model prevailing in all 12 countries with the exception of Georgia.

With regard to outpatient specialist care, there is a wider range of approaches within regions, in part due to differences in whether such care takes place in a separate clinic or in a hospital setting. Private clinics are the primary mode of provision in 14 OECD countries, while 8 rely on public hospitals and 2 on public centers. In western ECA, 5 countries use private centers, 8 use hospitals, and 4 rely on public centers. In eastern ECA, publicly provided outpatient specialist care is again the norm in all countries (either in polyclinics or in hospitals), with the exception of Georgia.

In the case of hospital ownership, there is far less diversity within and across regions. In brief, public hospitals are the predominant mode of delivery in all regions (figure 6.3). A minor caveat to this pattern is that OECD countries have a somewhat larger role for private nonprofit hospitals, which are relatively scarce in ECA countries. Out of over 50 countries surveyed, the only country in which for-profit hospitals account for a majority of acute-care beds is Georgia. But beyond the public-private mix, other important aspects of hospital management do differ across countries, as discussed below.

Thus, regarding the public-private mix in service delivery, the major difference between ECA (and more specifically the eastern part of the region) and OECD health systems is the stronger private orientation of primary care in the OECD. Both theory and evidence paint a mixed picture of the performance of public and private health providers (Hollingsworth 2008; Gaynor and Town 2012). This issue is revisited in the next section, with a focus on accountability.

Provider payment mechanisms have been another common focus of reform efforts in ECA during the past 20 years. The supply of medical care is very responsive to price, and the incentives created by the unit of payment—per day, per service, per person, retrospective, prospective, and so forth—can have a large impact on the quantity and quality of care provided. In general, fee-for-service (FFS) reimbursement may offer scope for better quality but at the risk of overprovision, while capitation and global budgets can help limit cost growth but providers may compromise on quality or overrefer patients to other facilities. Overall, provider payment is one of the most powerful tools available to policy makers for directing health care resources and implementing reform.

A wide range of provider payment approaches is applied across regions (figure 6.4). For primary care, 10 out of 24 OECD countries reimburse on a purely fee-for-service basis, while a further 7 use FFS in combination with another approach. The remaining seven

FIGURE 6.4

Regional Differences Are Larger with Respect to Payment of Primary Care than to Hospitals

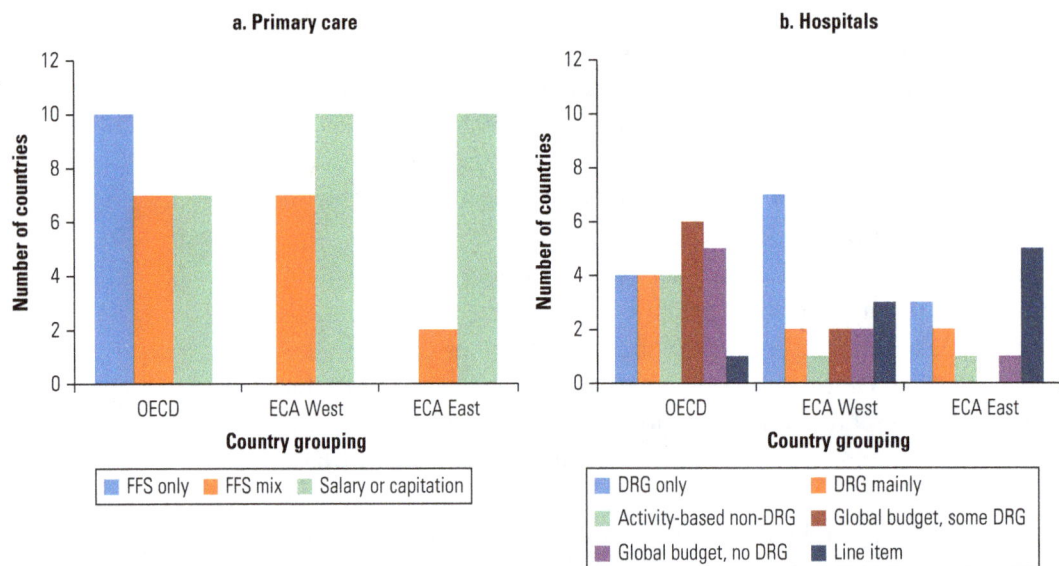

a. Primary care

b. Hospitals

Sources: Paris, Devaux, and Wei 2010; World Bank 2012.
Note: Figure shows provider payment methods. ECA = Europe and Central Asia; OECD = Organisation for Economic Co-operation and Development; FFS = fee for service; DRG = diagnosis-related group.

countries use either a capitation or a salary model or a combination of the two. Again, this group comprises mainly Mediterranean or Scandinavian countries: Greece, Iceland, Mexico, Portugal, Spain, Sweden, and Turkey. But Sweden has started to expand FFS payments in recent years.

In the western part of ECA, no country relies on a purely FFS model. Just under half use a mixed FFS system, while most have either capitation or salary-based payment. However, most countries in this region have some pay-for-performance scheme, in fact, more so than in the OECD. In eastern ECA, only Armenia and the Kyrgyz Republic have some FFS-based payment, while all others use capitation or salary.

Fewer cross-regional patterns are apparent with respect to hospital payment methods. In the OECD, about half the countries use predominantly diagnosis-related groups or other activity-based budgets, while the other half rely on global budgets (although these include a DRG element in some cases). In western ECA, the most common approach is DRGs, but again there are several countries using global budgets without an activity-based component, and three still use line-item budgeting (Albania, Montenegro, and Serbia). In eastern ECA, there is a growing use of DRGs but still a line-item approach in a significant number of countries.

Overall, ECA countries continue to use payment methods based on capitation or salary at primary care and line-item budgeting at the hospital level to a significantly greater degree than the OECD countries. This issue will be revisited with a focus on accountability in the next section.

Patient Pathways: A Trend toward Choice within Limits

Allowing more patient choice can promote competition in provision of health care by encouraging higher-quality services and potentially lower costs. However, patient choice needs to be balanced with concerns about the rational use of care and the pitfalls that may arise when patients bypass lower levels of care. As indicated in figure 6.5, in 18 of 24 OECD countries, the population is allowed to choose its primary care provider (in 3 of the 18, however, there are incentives to make certain choices). The exceptions are Denmark, Finland, Mexico, Portugal, Spain, and the United Kingdom. In the western part of ECA, all countries allow patient choice for primary care, while farther east, more countries limit choice. Similar regional patterns are present for choice of outpatient specialist care and hospital use.

FIGURE 6.5

A Trend toward Patient Choice but Less Consensus on Gate Keeping

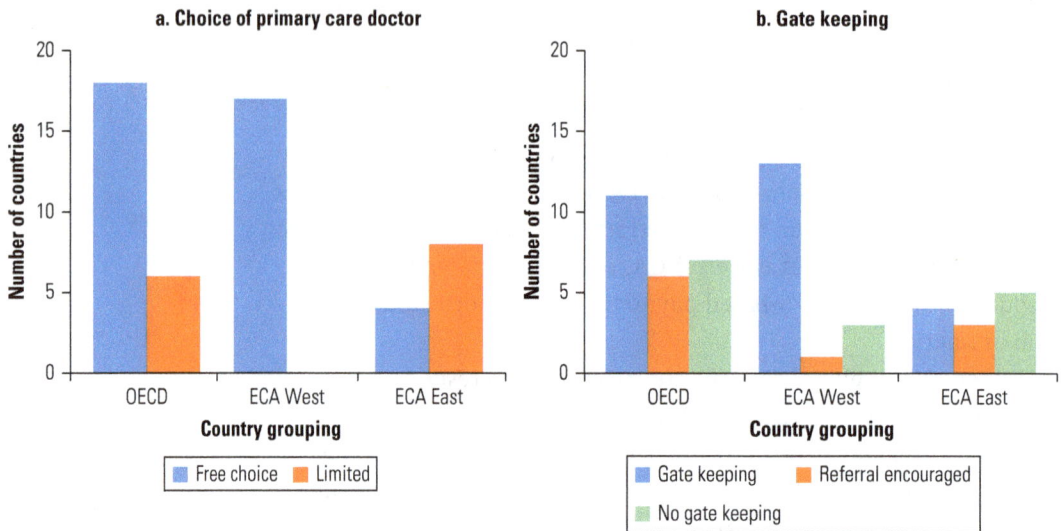

Sources: Paris, Devaux, and Wei 2010; World Bank 2012.
Note: ECA = Europe and Central Asia; OECD = Organisation for Economic Co-operation and Development.

There are fewer consistent regional patterns with regard to gate keeping for access to secondary care. In the OECD, nearly half the countries impose gate-keeping requirements, while a significant number also provide incentives to seek a referral, but seven countries have no obligation and no incentive to do so. In western ECA, nearly all countries have a gate-keeping requirement, while in eastern ECA all three approaches are used.

On other topics, there are fewer differences between OECD and ECA, at least on paper. This is true, for example, with respect to the regulation of physician and infrastructure supply. Differences are relatively minor: OECD countries are more likely to have quotas for medical students, and the OECD and western ECA are more likely than eastern ECA to have policies to address perceived doctor shortages. A majority of countries in all regions do not regulate practice location but do have policies to address maldistribution (for example, between urban and rural areas). In all regions, regional or central governments are typically involved in decisions about capacity planning for new hospitals, changes in bed supply, and provision of specific services. In the OECD, it is somewhat less common for governments to be involved in decisions about the supply of high-cost medical equipment compared to ECA.

This general overview provides only a glimpse of how different health systems are organized. Many have mixed approaches, and there are exceptions to many rules. As always, the same policy can be well implemented in one setting and poorly in another: the devil is often in the details. But in general, we now have some sense of where ECA health systems stand vis-à-vis advanced-country comparators.

To summarize, on financing, ECA is "more different" in coverage than in institutional design, which in any event differs widely across the OECD. With respect to facility ownership and provider payment issues, ECA looks more similar to OECD countries in the hospital sector than in primary care. Most countries in all regions have public hospitals, but these are paid through a wide range of methods, while in the case of primary care, public facilities with salaried doctors are far more common in eastern ECA than in the OECD. Patient pathways are somewhat less flexible in some ECA countries. Overall, health systems in the eastern part of ECA are "more different" from OECD counterparts than those in western ECA. We now turn to how this complex picture might translate into a policy agenda.

Ingredients, Not Recipes, for Successful Health Reform

The wide range of institutional characteristics in the health systems across the OECD (and ECA), as revealed by the stock-taking exercise of the previous section, points to the difficulty of identifying a "gold standard" health system. Of course, strong human resources and well-equipped facilities are essential, but health systems are defined by much more than just inputs. But there is too much cross-country diversity among successful health systems to pinpoint a single "right" policy mix to guide the implementation of health sector reform. So how can we move this agenda forward?

The challenge of identifying a reform agenda for health has similarities with long-standing debates about how to achieve economic growth. Indeed, improving population health and achieving higher growth rates arguably have much in common. They both involve complex, multisectoral "production functions" that change significantly according to the level of development. Institutional strengthening, overcoming behavioral norms, and technology adoption all figure prominently for both improving health and igniting growth. And in both cases, empirical work on cross-country determinants is hindered by a limited number of data points (countries) with which to analyze an abundance of possible theories. Thus, debates are more often informed by ideology than evidence.

Recent narratives concerned with the study of economic growth offer potential lessons for developing a health reform agenda. The Commission on Growth and Development (2008), which was tasked with taking stock of the state of knowledge on economic growth with a view toward deriving policy implications, arrived at the conclusion that it could propose "ingredients" but not "recipes." That is, it could identify certain common characteristics of countries with a strong track record of growth but not a fully articulated growth strategy (which would require specifying the quantities and sequencing of various measures), because "no single recipe exists." Moreover, the commission could not say if its list of ingredients is sufficient or whether they are all necessary. It was also believed that the appropriate model changes over time. The five main ingredients of economic growth identified by the Growth Commission based on success stories of the past were the following: (1) they fully exploited the world economy; (2) they let markets allocate resources; (3) they mustered high rates of saving and investment; (4) they maintained macroeconomic stability; and (5) they had committed, credible, and capable governments.

What, then, are the ingredients of successful health systems? Transposing the approach of the Growth Commission to the health reform arena, this section builds on the stock-taking exercise above and attempts to identify the most important inputs to health system reform. It identifies five key ingredients for health reform.

Three Ingredients for Accountable Health Systems: Payment, Autonomy, and Information

The first three ingredients of successful health systems that we identify here are as follows: (1) some element of activity-based payment; (2) provider autonomy; and (3) information for decision making. Before we describe each in turn, it is worth emphasizing from the outset that the overriding theme linking all three is *accountability*. Later on, we also highlight two additional ingredients: adequate risk pooling and leadership commitment.

The first ingredient is some degree of activity-based reimbursement, or "payment follows the patient." For primary care, activity-based reimbursement means some use of fee-for-service methods, even if only partially in the form of a mixed system with other approaches. It could also take the form of a pay-for-performance scheme. An important complement to activity-based payment is patient choice, allowing the population to "vote with its feet" away from low-quality providers in favor of better ones. The antithesis would be the payment of primary care in the form of a salary alone or, somewhat less problematic, using capitation (which can represent a logical transition step when purchasing capacity is underdeveloped), especially if it is not accompanied by patient choice.

For hospitals, activity-based payment is increasingly taking the form of diagnosis-related groups in OECD countries, and many countries in ECA have started to move in this direction. Other fee-for-service approaches are possible, as are mixed methods of payment, whereby activity-based reimbursement is combined with other approaches. In the hospital setting, the absence of this ingredient would be represented by line-item budgeting, or pure global budgeting, both of which are increasingly rare in the OECD but endure in parts of ECA. Note that this ingredient refers to how hospitals are paid, not the doctors who work in them, most of whom are paid by salary in all regions.

Activity-based payment mechanisms are highlighted as a key ingredient of successful health systems due to the signal they send to providers of medical care: that services for patients are their core responsibility and thus the basis on which they will be paid. It strengthens incentives to provide the necessary medical services to patients and to be responsive to their needs; in its absence, providers are more likely to neglect their responsibilities. It is not that pecuniary self-interest is the only thing that motivates doctors; indeed, there is ample evidence that nonmonetary factors matter, too. In addition, payment mechanisms need to be mindful of efficiency considerations, and thus open-ended, retrospective fee-for-service reimbursement of all costs is not a viable solution. But the nature of primary care provision is somewhat self-limiting, and at hospitals, the DRG method pays prospectively for patients based on diagnosis upon admission, not retrospectively for all services rendered.

In the OECD, only Iceland, Mexico, Portugal, and Spain have neither FFS payment for primary care nor some DRG or activity-based component for hospitals. The basic trend in the OECD is also moving toward more of this ingredient at primary care, such as reforms over the past 20 years in Finland, Sweden, and the United Kingdom, which have historically had a more publicly integrated model of finance and provision. Meanwhile, about half the countries in eastern ECA have no payment following the patient in either the primary care or the hospital setting. While it might be argued that paying salaries is the only administratively feasible option in low-income settings, most if not all of ECA is beyond that stage. Strong purchasing capacity cannot be achieved overnight, but making steady progress will be important.

The second ingredient is provider autonomy. It has been defined as the extent of the "decision rights" that facilities have over the many and varied aspects of producing health care services. These include decisions over labor and capital inputs, output level and mix, and management processes, among others (Preker and Harding 2003). Provider autonomy is particularly important in the hospital setting, where decision making is more complex. Historically, much of ECA had almost no autonomy: facilities were essentially integrated units of the ministry of health. Line-item hospital budgeting, which persists in several ECA countries, is in many ways the antithesis of autonomy: how and how much can be spent is preordained by central authorities.

In the OECD, provider autonomy is typically achieved for primary care in the form of private solo or group practices. In eastern ECA, public primary care provision continues to predominate, as shown above. In the hospital setting, the differences between OECD countries and ECA with regard to provider autonomy are particularly apparent in whether hospital managers have complete autonomy for the recruitment of medical staff and other health professionals or if the central or local government decides. Over two-thirds of OECD health systems extend this autonomy. The exceptions are France, Greece, Ireland, Italy, Mexico, Norway, and Spain. About half the countries in western ECA have that same degree of hospital autonomy, with the exceptions primarily in the countries of the former Yugoslavia and Turkey. In eastern ECA, only Armenia, Georgia, and the Kyrgyz Republic allow hospitals to make those decisions. Hospital managers in the OECD are also more likely to have autonomy over the remuneration of medical staff, although to a lesser extent than for recruitment. As noted, there is somewhat more latitude for OECD hospitals to make decisions related to high-cost equipment, but otherwise there is less autonomy in infrastructure planning across all regions, in part reflecting concerns about overinvestment.

A shift toward hospital autonomy has been observed across advanced European health systems in recent years (Chevalier, Garel, and Levitan 2009; Saltman, Duran, and Dubois 2011). These have taken many different forms, and various terms are used to describe them—foundation trusts, public joint-stock companies, and so on—but the unifying factor has been greater autonomy.

Provider payment and autonomy work best hand in hand. Creating payment-based incentives without the decision-making power to act on them is likely to fall short of achieving intended objectives. Figure 6.6 looks at this issue in the context of primary care. Only three OECD countries—Mexico, Portugal, and Spain—have no

FIGURE 6.6

Accountability of Primary Care Is Stronger in the OECD than in ECA

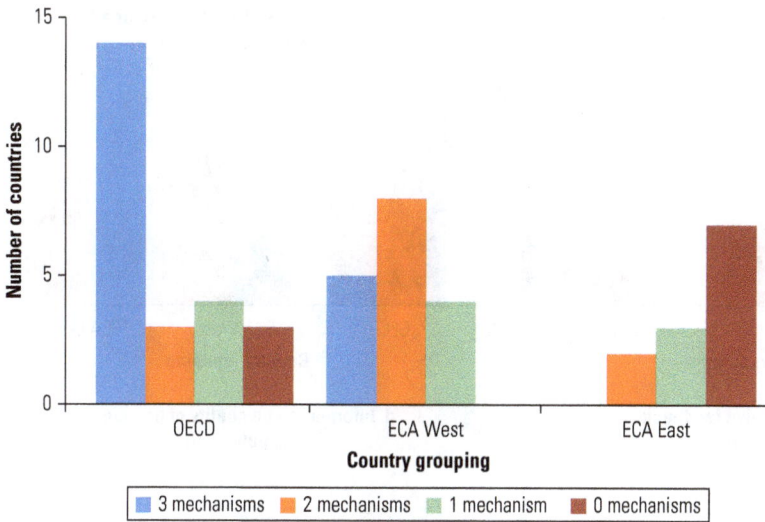

Sources: Paris, Devaux, and Wei 2010; World Bank 2012.
Note: Figure shows the number of primary care accountability mechanisms: activity-based payment, provider choice, and autonomy for primary care. ECA = Europe and Central Asia; OECD = Organisation for Economic Co-operation and Development.

element of fee-for-service payment, no patient choice, and publicly provided primary care (that is, limited autonomy). Over three-quarters of the OECD and western ECA have at least two of three. Meanwhile, about half the countries in the eastern part of ECA have this model, and only two—Armenia and the Kyrgyz Republic—have at least two out of three. Mismatches in payment methods and autonomy (or lack thereof) have also been a common problem in the hospital sector in many ECA countries (Jakab, Preker, and Harding 2003).

The pattern of payment and autonomy arrangements for primary care in ECA represent a key potential explanation for the weakness in primary care delivery (including control of cardiovascular risk factors) described in chapter 3. Reforms in this area could be a first step toward improving outcomes.

The third ingredient is the use of information for decision making. Health systems produce a wide array of "products," and at any point in time there is likely to be significant variation in performance across services and providers. The availability of information flows to monitor and act upon this variation is important for ongoing system improvement. In which region is disease incidence rising or falling the most? Which physicians prescribe more antibiotics or refer more patients than their colleagues? Which hospitals have the lowest

FIGURE 6.7

Greater Use of Information in OECD Health Systems than in ECA

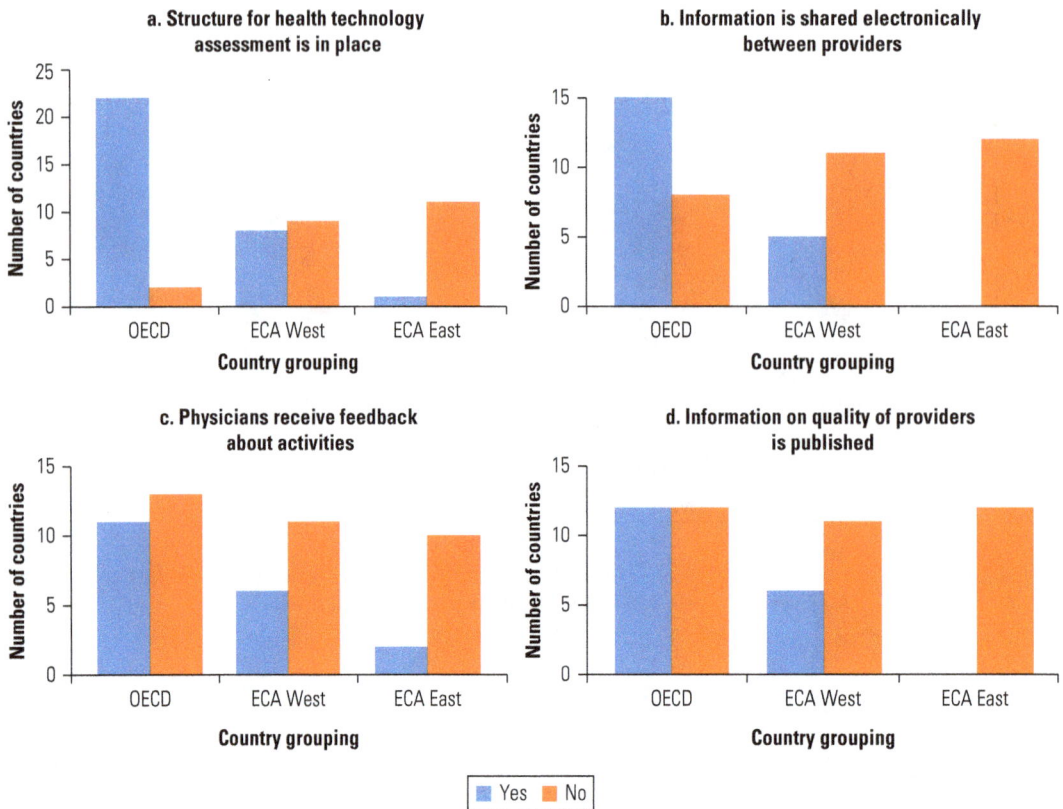

a. Structure for health technology assessment is in place

b. Information is shared electronically between providers

c. Physicians receive feedback about activities

d. Information on quality of providers is published

■ Yes   ■ No

Sources: Paris, Devaux, and Wei 2010; World Bank 2012.
Note: ECA = Europe and Central Asia; OECD = Organisation for Economic Co-operation and Development.

mortality rates for patients admitted with stroke? Answering these questions and acting on the information is important. In essence, it is a health system analog to operational research by businesses. This ingredient also reinforces the importance of having some activity-based payment methods: salaries and global budgeting yield no information about services provided.

Figure 6.7 illustrates the differences across the OECD and ECA with respect to several examples of health system use of information. These examples are whether there is any use of health technology assessment to determine whether a service should be covered; whether providers share information electronically, which can strengthen coordination of care and reduce duplicative and wasteful care; whether physicians receive feedback about their activities, which can promote continuous performance improvement; and whether information is published on the quality of individual providers, which can help patients make decisions about where to seek care and provides an incentive for better quality of care. Individually, these measures are not uniformly used across the OECD, but the tendency is in that direction. In eastern ECA, these information tools are almost nonexistent. A related ingredient is analytical expertise and institutional structures (for example, health information centers) that can maximize the use of this information. Some ECA countries have invested in these areas, but much remains to be done.

As noted, the unifying theme of these three ingredients for successful health systems is the concept of accountability. This concept has been defined as both "answerability" and sanctions and has been divided into financial, performance, and political accountability (Brinkerhoff 2004). Thus, payment that follows the patient helps signal what providers are accountable for; autonomy affords them the ability to make decisions for themselves as they seek to fulfill their responsibilities; and information flows generate the necessary data for "asking questions," assessing their performance, and taking action (or not), accordingly.

An additional channel for improving accountability is through mechanisms that promote patient rights. The stock-taking exercise described in the previous section revealed that most countries in all regions have adopted some measures with this objective. These may include a formal definition of patient rights in legislation or elsewhere, complaint desks at hospitals, or an ombudsman. But there is sometimes a wide gap between the de jure and the de facto patient empowerment afforded by these mechanisms, with potential channels for asserting rights typically less meaningful in eastern regions of ECA than in the OECD.

Two Additional Ingredients: Adequate Risk Pooling and Committed Leadership

In addition to the three ingredients for accountable institutions already noted, it is also worth highlighting two others that are required for successful health reform. The first is adequate risk pooling. No health system, regardless of how well its institutions correspond to those prevailing in advanced countries, will be able to achieve key system objectives if risk-pooling arrangements are inadequate and fragmented. The counterfactual—a high reliance on OOP spending—can be self-defeating in the pursuit of health reform. Health financing institutions that ensure adequate risk pooling are not only important for financial protection and equity but also for helping create the conditions for stronger purchasing power and regulatory authority.

The final ingredient, which is borrowed directly from the list developed by the Growth Commission, is "committed, capable, and credible governments." In part, this ingredient encompasses the concept of stewardship for the health system, including with regard to human resources, disease management, capacity planning, surveillance, and so on. But it is much more than that. Successful reform requires vision and leadership. It means taking on vested interests, whether in the medical establishment, political actors, or elsewhere in society, to usher in new reforms that will help achieve sectoral objectives. That necessity is arguably true, particularly in public health. The difference between being five years ahead of the curve and five years behind the curve in tobacco control, for example, is a decade of lives lost to preventable disease. The experience of Turkey in this regard was highlighted in chapter 3.

In sum, we have identified five major ingredients of successful reform experiences and health systems. These are payment that follows the patient, provider autonomy, information for decision making, adequate risk pooling, and leadership. They all amount to what might be termed "macro" health reforms; in previous chapters, we explored some of the "micro" reforms (for example, specific regulations or changes to a benefit package) that can contribute to specific objectives.

If those ECA countries that lag behind can make progress on this institutional reform agenda, it should help produce more rapid convergence of key sectoral performance indicators with those prevailing in the EU-15 and OECD. But ultimately each country will need to combine these ingredients in different ways and at different points in time to develop its own "recipe" for health reform.

References

Borowitz, M., and R. Atun. 2006. "The Unfinished Journey from Semashko to Bismarck: Health Reform in Central Asia from 1991 to 2006." *Central Asian Survey* 25 (4): 419–40.

Brinkerhoff, D.W. 2004. "Accountability and Health Systems: Toward Conceptual Clarity and Policy Relevance." *Health Policy and Planning* 19 (6): 371–79.

Chevalier, F., P. Garel, and J. Levitan. 2009. *Hospitals in the 27 Member States of the European Union*. Dexia: Paris.

Commission on Growth and Development. 2008. *The Growth Report: Strategies for Sustained Growth and Inclusive Development*. Washington, DC: World Bank.

Cutler, D. 2002. "Equality, Efficiency, and Market Fundamentals: The Dynamics of International Medical Care Reform." *Journal of Economic Literature* 40 (3): 881–906.

Cutler, D., and R. Zeckhauser, 2000. "The Anatomy of Health Insurance." In *Handbook of Health Economics,* Vol. 1, edited by A. Culyer and J. Newhouse, 563–643. Amsterdam: Elsevier BV.

Davis, C. 2010. "Understanding the Legacy: Health Financing Systems in the USSR and Central and Eastern Europe prior to Transition." In *Implementing Health Financing Reform: Lessons from Countries in Transition,* edited by J. Kutzin, C. Cashin, and M. Jakab, 25–64. Copenhagen: European Observatory.

Docteur, E., and H. Oxley. 2003. "Health-Care Systems: Lessons from the Reform Experience." Health Working Papers 9, Organisation for Economic Co-operation and Development, Paris.

Figueras, J., M. McKee, J. Cain, and S. Lessof, eds. 2004. *Health Systems in Transition: Learning from Experience.* Copenhagen: European Observatory.

Gaynor, M., and R. Town. 2012. "Competition in Health Care Markets." In *Handbook of Health Economics,* vol. 2, edited by Mark V. Pauly, Thomas G. McGuire, and Pedro P. Barros, 499–637. Oxford: Elsevier Science BV.

Hollingsworth, B. 2008. "The Measurement of Efficiency and Productivity of Health Care Delivery." *Health Economics* 17: 1107–28.

Jakab, M., A. Preker, and A. Harding. 2003. "The Missing Link? Hospital Reform in Transition Economies." In *Innovations in Health Service Delivery: The Corporatization of Public Hospitals,* edited by A. Preker and A. Harding, 207–38. Washington, DC: World Bank.

Kutzin, J., C. Cashin, and M. Jakab. 2010. *Implementing Health Financing Reform: Lessons from Countries in Transition.* Copenhagen: European Observatory.

Leiter, A. M., and E. Theurl. 2010. "The Convergence of Health Care Financing Structures: Empirical Evidence form OECD Countries." *European Journal of Health Economics* 13 (1): 7–18.

Maier, C. B., and J. M. Martin-Moreno. 2011. "Quo vadis SANEPID? A Cross-Country Analysis of Public Health Reforms in 10 Post-Soviet States." *Health Policy* 102 (1): 18–25.

Moreno-Serra, R., and A. Wagstaff. 2010. "System-Wide Impacts of Hospital Payment Reforms: Evidence from Central and Eastern Europe and Central Asia." *Journal of Health Economics* 29 (4): 585–602.

OECD (Organisation for Economic Co-operation and Development). 2010. "Health Care Systems: Efficiency and Institutions." Working Paper 769, OECD, Paris.

Paris, V., M. Devaux, and L. Wei. 2010. "Health System Institutional Characteristics: A Survey of 29 OECD Countries." Health Working Paper 50, OECD, Paris.

Preker, A., and A. Harding, eds. 2003. *Innovations in Health Service Delivery: The Corporatization of Public Hospitals.* Washington, DC: World Bank.

Rechel, B., and M. McKee. 2008. "Lessons from Polyclinics in Central and Eastern Europe." *British Medical Journal* 337: a952.

———. 2009. "Health Reform in Central and Eastern Europe and the Former Soviet Union." *Lancet* 374: 1186–95.

Rothgang, H. 2010. *The State and Healthcare: Comparing OECD Countries.* New York: Palgrave Macmillan.

Saltman, R. B., A. Duran, and H. Dubois. 2011. *Governing Public Hospitals: Reform Strategies and the Movement towards Institutional Autonomy.* Copenhagen: European Observatory.

Wagstaff, A. 2010. "Social Health Insurance Re-Examined." *Health Economics* 19 (5): 503–17.

Wagstaff, A., and R. Moreno-Serra. 2009. "Europe and Central Asia's Great Post-Communist Social Health Insurance Experiment: Aggregate Impacts on Health Sector Outcomes." *Journal of Health Economics* 28 (2): 322–40.

WHO. 2012. National Health Accounts (database), World Health Organization, Geneva, http://www.who.int/nha/expenditure_database/en.

World Bank. 2000. *ECA Health, Nutrition, and Population: A Decade of Experience.* Washington, DC: World Bank.

———. 2005. "Review of Experience of Family Medicine in Europe and Central Asia." Report No. 32354-ECA, World Bank, Washington, DC.

———. 2012. "Health System Institutional Characteristics in ECA." Draft. World Bank, Washington, DC.

CHAPTER 7

Summary Q&A

This chapter summarizes the main messages of the report in a question-and-answer format.

1. Why write a report on health in ECA?

The story of health in Europe and Central Asia (ECA) is in many respects a story of long-term underperformance on a fundamental aspect of development. Although life expectancy in the region as a whole is only slightly below average for its income level, the long-term trend has been weaker than in other regions. In the 1960s, the average lifespan in ECA was just 5 years less than in Western Europe, but 10 years more than in Latin America and 20 years more than in East Asia and the Middle East. But since then, the life expectancy gap with the EU-15 has widened significantly, while other regions have caught up and overtaken ECA.

A similar regional story could be told using many other health indicators, and there has also been a lack of convergence on key outcomes in health financing. However, it is not a uniform story across the region. Turkey has experienced very large health gains over this period, the Balkans have performed in line with global norms, and Central Europe has steadily improved since the 1990s. But many other countries have made much less progress. The reality of ECA's long-term health sector struggles is not new; but as the years go by, the policy urgency only increases. The slow progress of ECA's health outcomes is also of global significance. While there have been tremendous gains in health around the world over the past half-century, there have been two major exceptions: Sub-Saharan Africa, due to the HIV/AIDS epidemic, and Eastern Europe.

2. Among the many development challenges facing the region, is health really such a priority for the populations of ECA?

Yes. When survey respondents across the region were asked to identify their top priority for additional government investment, health was ranked as the first choice in about three-quarters of ECA countries, both in 2006 and in 2010. The result held true among both men and women, old and young, rich and poor. This sentiment is consistent with a body of economic research suggesting that better health is a major contributor to overall welfare improvement. People want to live long, healthy lives and are willing to forgo many other things to achieve it. For example, survey respondents in six ECA countries were about evenly divided when asked to choose, hypo-thetically, between living in a country with a European health system or in one with a European income level.

Moreover, the priority accorded to health is unlikely to be transi-tory, suggesting that it is a policy issue here to stay. As people become richer, they tend to devote an ever-larger share of their resources to achieving better health. Health was also a top priority for additional government investment in several Western European countries, and expectations for a prominent government role in the sector are higher than in other areas such as pensions and jobs. For all these reasons, the health sector is likely to figure more prominently as an election issue as well.

3. Shouldn't policy makers focus on economic growth, and better health will follow?

Economic growth is vital to ECA's long-term prosperity and for poverty reduction and will also be a key enabler of allocating more resources to health. But growth does not automatically produce better health. Average growth of gross domestic product (GDP) has been higher in ECA than in the EU-15 since the mid-1990s, but despite progress with income convergence, the long-term divergence of health outcomes has not been reversed. In fact, the global experi-ence does not suggest that economic growth will inevitably lead to better health, as there has been very little correlation between changes in real GDP and life expectancy around the world over the past 50 years. Instead, the major driver of improved health outcomes in middle- and high-income countries is the expanded application of health-improving knowledge and technology to both personal behavior and medical care. Concerted public action to improve health systems is a necessary condition for improving health outcomes.

4. What are the main health problems in the region?

Cardiovascular disease is the major health problem in ECA. Health outcomes in ECA have fallen behind those of the EU-15 in large part because the region has yet to achieve the "cardiovascular revolution" that has taken place in the West over the past 50 years. Circulatory diseases account for over half the life expectancy gap between ECA and the EU-15 today, and better cardiovascular outcomes were also responsible for over half the health gains in the EU-15 in recent decades. The predominance of a single disease group represents an obvious target for policy action. The progress made against heart disease is where the miracle of modern medicine has been most evident, but many countries in ECA have yet to fully seize this potential.

In addition, two other factors behind the life expectancy gap also stand out. The first is neonatal mortality (that is, death within the first 28 days of life), which accounts for the majority of deaths before age one. The second is external causes, mainly due to alcohol-related road traffic injuries, which are responsible for an extraordinary and unnecessary loss of life concentrated among the working-age male population in a relatively small number of countries in the region. More broadly, other important priorities include the unfinished agenda of the Millennium Development Goals (especially goals related to HIV/AIDS and tuberculosis), the growing challenge of cancer, and major sources of morbidity such as mental health.

5. What should be done to address cardiovascular disease and other health priorities?

The experience of more advanced health systems suggests that both prevention and treatment must play a central role in ECA's future health agenda. The starting point for reducing cardiovascular disease mortality is to address its major risk factors in the general population, before individuals need medical care. Among the most important of these are tobacco and alcohol use. Men in ECA smoke more than their counterparts in almost any other region and significantly more than in the EU-15. Alcohol use—in particular, binge drinking—is also a major problem in some countries. The most effective tobacco control policy is to increase cigarette taxes, but in many countries, tax rates remain quite low. Smoking bans in public places could also be more widely introduced. Across the region, there is widespread support for public health measures to help address tobacco and alcohol use, especially among women. But while there are exceptions, in many countries the policies lag behind, suggesting that public opinion is ahead of government action.

Addressing cardiovascular disease will also require better management of risk factors such as high blood pressure and cholesterol in the primary care setting. Only about 10 percent of those with hypertension in many ECA countries have it under control, compared to over 50 percent in some advanced health systems. People are also less likely to be tested for high cholesterol. Various policy measures can help improve the management of these risk factors through primary care. These may include efforts to improve access and affordability of outpatient drugs by including them in benefit packages, disease management programs, and, potentially, reimbursement of providers through pay-for-performance schemes that better incentivize attention to risk factors.

Last, while the emphasis should be on efforts to prevent illness and manage risk factors, health systems must also aim to achieve a high quality of care in the treatment of chronic and acute episodes of illness. Better management of heart attacks, strokes, and neonatal conditions has been a major factor behind health gains in the West, but survey evidence from ECA suggests there is significant room for improvement in the region. A range of interventions can help improve quality of care, including stronger hospital management practices and performance measurement linked to payment, professional recognition, and peer review. Those health system–strengthening measures for addressing cardiovascular disease will also benefit other causes of ill health in the region. Overall, many of the services that have proven so important in the health advances achieved elsewhere—from cancer screening to the treatment of depression—are not yet being provided on an adequate scale across much of the ECA region.

6. Will closing the life expectancy gap be expensive?

Closing a large share of the life expectancy gap between ECA and the EU-15 does not need to be expensive. Higher tobacco taxes would in fact generate additional revenues. Generic drugs to treat cardiovascular risk factors through primary care can cost as little as a few dollars per patient per month. Both of these interventions are among the most cost effective available. In general, between public health legislation and managing risk factors through primary care, there are major cardiovascular health gains available for very low cost. A big part of the life expectancy gap—probably at least two-thirds and perhaps more—can be addressed through lower levels of care. The majority of potential health improvements will not involve hospitals; yet these absorb undue attention and resources.

There are, however, some interventions that have contributed substantially to improved health in the West that do not come as cheaply: for example, certain heart procedures such as angioplasty and bypass operations, some neonatal technologies, and wider access to cancer screening and treatment. Countries will need to make careful choices about what can be afforded.

7. How can the growing demand for medical care be financed?

Both in ECA and around the world, health financing is drawn largely from household out-of-pocket (OOP) sources or from the government budget (that is, through tax revenues, including mandatory social health insurance). The growing demand for health care must therefore be financed without imposing an undue burden on either source. Too much OOP spending for health care is a concern because it can undermine financial protection or equity, or both. That is, OOP spending may be "catastrophic" (exceeding some significant threshold of total household expenditures) or "impoverishing" (if it pushes some households below the poverty line). OOP spending can also pose an important barrier to health care, resulting in significant inequalities in utilization between rich and poor. But an excessive burden of health spending on the government budget can be wasteful and pose a threat to fiscal sustainability.

Currently, the relative importance of OOP spending and government budget sources varies widely across the region. This picture has not changed significantly over time, as very few countries in ECA have significantly reduced their reliance on OOP spending since 1997. As a result, inadequate financial protection remains a problem in about half the ECA region. The objective should not be to lower OOP spending to zero, but theory and evidence suggest that less than 25 percent of total health financing drawn from this source is a reasonable policy objective.

8. What can be done to make health financing systems in ECA more pro-poor?

The major priority for making health financing systems more pro-poor is to reduce the out-of-pocket payments people face at the point of care. In many ECA countries, households spend on average more than twice as much on health, measured as a share of their total expenditures, as their counterparts in the EU-15. A large proportion of this spending is on drugs, and much of it is catastrophic. Household survey data from across the region show that the more heavily a country relies on OOP spending for health financing, the more common these catastrophic episodes become, the greater the inequality is in use of care across socioeconomic groups, and the more people fall into poverty as a result of their medical bills. In about 10 ECA countries, the share of households facing catastrophic health care episodes is twice as high as in the EU-15.

In some countries—especially those with small health budgets—a necessary step toward strengthening financial protection is through more government health spending. This step may require expanding the benefit package, for example, by including some outpatient drugs, or it may mean better coverage of specific populations, such as those working in the informal sector or the Roma population in some countries of Central and Eastern Europe. In brief, special effort should be made to ensure that improvements in financial protection and access to care benefit the poorest first, through targeted health programs. Georgia offers a successful example of using a proxy means test to target additional health resources to the poor. But bigger budgets are not the only issue. Rent seeking by health care providers in the form of informal payments and high pharmaceutical price markups are also important causes of weak financial protection in ECA.

9. Are ECA countries spending too much on health by global standards?

No. Health spending in the region is generally in line with global patterns, given the region's income level and age structure. In fact, health budgets in ECA have increased more slowly in recent years than in Western Europe, East Asia, and Latin America. In general, moderate growth in health spending as a share of GDP is to be expected in middle- and high-income countries and should not be a cause for concern as long as it is translated into improved outcomes instead of more waste.

While there is naturally a lot of concern about the growing cost of health budgets, passing judgment on any policy or program requires some effort to consider the benefits, too. As countries grow richer and basic needs are met, the importance of health in individual preferences becomes even greater. Living longer, healthier lives is preferred to compressing more consumption into a fixed life span. For this reason, long-term growth in health spending in advanced countries has on the whole been worth it, even in the presence of significant waste, due to the high value attached to health gains achieved through medical advances. The major policy challenge is that while health systems at their best can provide life-saving care, they also often have a large amount of waste. The policy imperative is to cut one without cutting the other.

10. What are the main sources of waste, and how should these be addressed?

Excess hospital infrastructure and inefficient spending on pharmaceuticals are both major sources of waste. There are nearly twice as many hospitals per person in the Commonwealth of Independent States region as in the EU-15. The result is high fixed costs, unnecessarily long admissions, and hospital beds that are occupied for the wrong reasons: for example, in many ECA countries, people are far more likely to be hospitalized for hypertension than in the EU-15, a condition that should be controlled at lower levels of care. Often, the major constraint to reducing hospital capacity is political will, but there are countries in the region, such as Estonia, that have successfully made these reforms. Ultimately, it is in the interest of the health system and patients alike for a population to spend less rather than more time in hospital.

With regard to pharmaceuticals, governments across the region are struggling to contain the pressure that these exert on their budgets. One challenge is high prices. In many countries, there is scope for procurement reform and for more "smart purchasing" of drugs. This may include a preference for generics, price regulation, and innovative contracting approaches. Another problem is overconsumption, for which both providers and patients bear some responsibility. Clear treatment protocols, drug lists, and generic promotion can help.

A significant and sometimes overlooked part of the agenda for cutting back on waste is not about pursuing major systemic reforms but rather about understanding why, for example, some doctors refer more patients to higher levels of care, order more diagnostic procedures, or prescribe more drugs than their colleagues. The same applies to why some hospitals have higher readmission rates or higher mortality rates for specific types of care than others. The organizations that pay for services should keep track of these patterns and make use of this information to address the outliers through more active approaches to purchasing care. Investing in the analytical capacity to fulfill this role can play a key part in setting the stage for efficiency gains.

11. Is there an ideal health system design that ECA should adopt?

It is not possible to identify an "ideal" health system on the basis of experiences of advanced countries such as those in the Organisation for Economic Co-operation and Development (OECD). There is considerable heterogeneity that exists among them, but there are also some common tendencies. As a result, it is possible to identify "ingredients" but not "recipes" for institutional reform of health systems. In other words, it is possible to identify certain common characteristics of countries with strong health systems but not a fully articulated model (which would require specifying the quantities and sequencing of various measures), because no single recipe exists. Several of these ingredients are closely tied to the concept of accountability in service provision.

12. What institutional reforms need to be undertaken in ECA?

Five key ingredients are proposed for the institutional reform agenda of ECA's health systems. Although not universal among OECD countries, these ingredients are widespread and are becoming more so.

The first is some degree of activity-based reimbursement, or "payment follows the patient." This form of reimbursement implies at least a partial use of fee-for-service and case-based payments—not salaries and line-item budgets. The second ingredient is provider autonomy, or the extent to which a facility has "decision rights" over the many aspects of producing health care services. In the OECD, such autonomy is typically achieved through private solo or group practices for primary care and considerable autonomy for hospital managers in areas such as the recruitment of their health workforce. The third ingredient is the use of information for decision making. Health systems produce thousands of individual services at hundreds of different facilities on a daily basis, and there is likely to be significant variation in performance across both these dimensions. The availability of information flows to monitor and act on this variation is important for ongoing system improvement.

The fourth ingredient is adequate risk pooling. The health financing policy agenda for ECA is chiefly to expand coverage of people and services through adequate risk pooling, with more than a single feasible institutional approach available for doing so. No health system will be able to achieve key system objectives if health financing relies primarily on small, fragmented risk pools and OOP spending. The final ingredient to moving the health reform agenda forward is committed, credible leadership. Vested interests will need to be overcome, but there is popular demand for stronger health systems across the region.

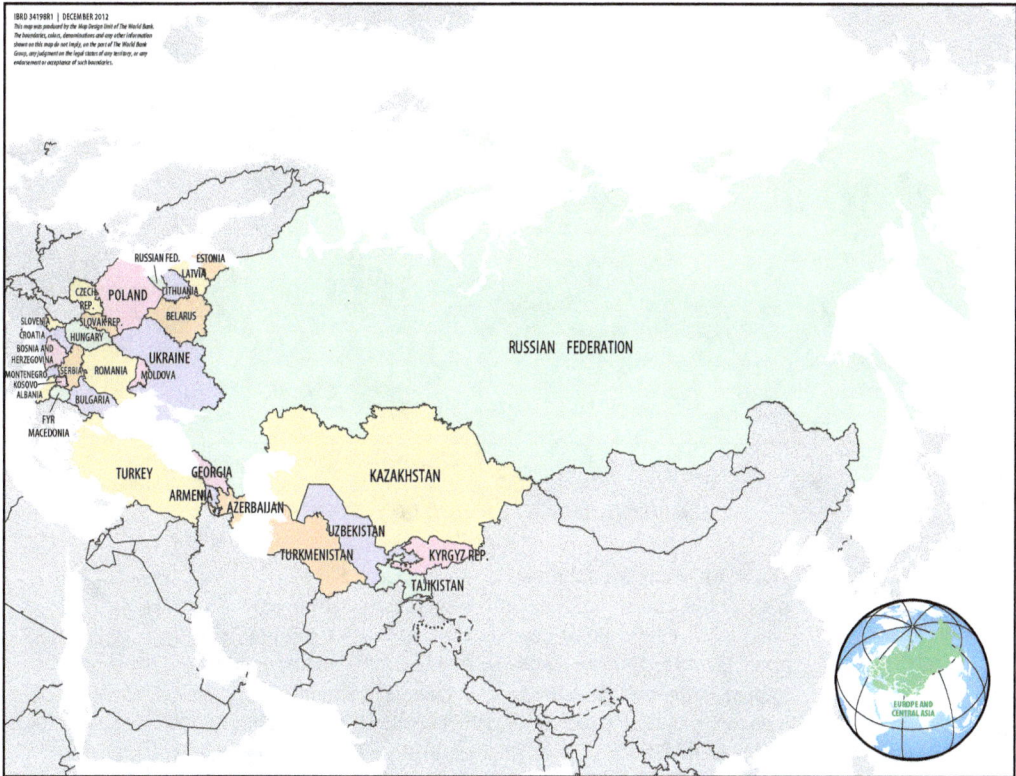

IBRD 34199R1 | DECEMBER 2012
This map was produced by the Map Design Unit of The World Bank.
The boundaries, colors, denominations and any other information
shown on this map do not imply, on the part of The World Bank
Group, any judgment on the legal status of any territory, or any
endorsement or acceptance of such boundaries.

This report is part of a series undertaken by the Europe and Central Asia Region of the World Bank.
Earlier reports have investigated poverty, jobs, trade, migration, demography, and productivity growth.
The series covers the following countries:

Albania	Latvia
Armenia	Lithuania
Azerbaijan	Moldova
Belarus	Montenegro
Bosnia and Herzegovina	Poland
Bulgaria	Romania
Croatia	Russian Federation
Czech Republic	Serbia
Estonia	Slovak Republic
FYR Macedonia	Slovenia
Georgia	Tajikistan
Hungary	Turkey
Kazakhstan	Turkmenistan
Kosovo	Ukraine
Kyrgyz Republic	Uzbekistan

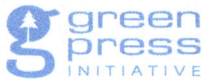

www.ingramcontent.com/pod-product-compliance
Lightning Source LLC
Chambersburg PA
CBHW081645280326
41928CB00069B/2995